The Politics of Disability

A Need for a Just Society Inclusive of People with Disabilities

by

Peter Gibilisco

Foreword by
Frank Stilwell

CCB Publishing
British Columbia, Canada

The Politics of Disability:
A Need for a Just Society Inclusive of People with Disabilities

Copyright ©2014 by Peter Gibilisco
ISBN-13   978-1-77143-155-2
First Edition

Library and Archives Canada Cataloguing in Publication
Gibilisco, Peter, 1962-, author
The politics of disability : a need for a just society inclusive of people with disabili-
ties / written by Peter Gibilisco, foreword by Frank Stilwell. -- First edition.
Issued in print and electronic formats.
ISBN 978-1-77143-155-2 (pbk.).--ISBN 978-1-77143-156-9 (pdf)
Additional cataloguing data available from Library and Archives Canada

Cover artwork: Photo of Peter Gibilisco courtesy of Michael Silver

Publisher: CCB Publishing
             British Columbia, Canada
             www.ccbpublishing.com

Contents

PREFACE

I wrote this book because my previous one sold at a ridiculously expensive price making it beyond the reach of many within the disability sector. For me, the task was daunting, but, in the long run, very satisfying. Knowing that there may be many of you who may find my thoughts valuable and motivating is what made me focus and strive to achieve my goal.

There is not a great deal of demand for publishing works about disability, and consequently many Australian and worldwide publishing houses rejected my manuscript. Therefore, this suggests to me the importance of working to strengthen the disability sector; there is a large population in this sector who lack a strong voice. I believe that this book will be a wake-up call to many within and without the disability sector to actively engage and address prevalent issues.

I faced moments of emotional trauma and disappointments while writing my book. These feelings were heightened because of the nature of my disability, and this was a hurdle I needed to overcome. As is the case for many of us with a disability, life at times has not been fair to me, but I believe there is hope, and I will continue to fight.

The progressive nature of my disability has got to such a stage that, unfortunately, my typing speed is extremely slow, and it has made my ability to perform certain keystrokes increasingly difficult. I have spent much more than 10 times writing this book compared to what an average writer would do. I have persevered and achieved my goal spurred on by the thought that I am fighting for justice, and the belief that I can make a difference.

ACKNOWLEDGEMENTS

There are many people I wish to thank, so please don't be offended if I forget someone. All of these people have assisted me a great deal in putting my thoughts into words.

First, I would like to mention Amanda Gunawardena, my academic support worker, who helped me with typing, editing and all administrative duties, and without whom I could not have achieved this.

My gratitude goes out to Susan Prior who helped me immensely by editing my book.

To Debbie Mackenzie and Suzette Diaz, both long-term support workers who hold a special place in my heart.

Thanks for this book also go out to Paul Rabinovitch of CCB Publishing who made my dream achievable. I really needed his guidance and assistance regarding administrative issues related to the publishing process.

Thank you my friend Peter Sember for your contribution to my book, and also your friendship that kept me going when times got tough.

I would also like to acknowledge the assistance by my two support workers, Cunxia Li and Ajay Joseph, who shared their valuable knowledge and thoughts.

My sincere gratitude goes to Richard Dent whose valuable knowledge made a large contribution to my book.

I wish to acknowledge the support of Tharuka Bodaragama whose assistance with my academic support work was invaluable.

I would also like to thank my family for being there for me through thick and thin. This book goes out especially to my mother, whom I know would have been proud of me.

This book is dedicated to four men who have each been an inspiration for my academic work: Hugh Stretton for his encouragement, inspiration and needed help. Bruce Wearne who has always been there, and assisted and encouraged me with my writing. Frank Stilwell whose knowledge has helped me mould my book into something better. And, Tim Marjoribanks who has been a major influence on this book and, in fact, all my work over the years.

FOREWORD

Frank Stilwell, Professor Emeritus in Political Economy, University of Sydney

'The personal is the political' is an adage most commonly associated with feminism. This book shows that it is equally applicable to people with disabilities. Personal struggles to cope with the difficulties of day-to-day existence are linked with broader political challenges to foster greater empathy in public attitudes and create improved public policies.

Most people would agree with the goal of creating a fair society, although they interpret the challenge rather differently. Some say it requires narrowing the gap in income and wealth that divides rich and poor people. Maybe a wide-ranging assault on 'class' is needed. At a bare minimum, the eradication of poverty is a central element in genuine social progress. So, too, is creating equality of opportunity. Indeed, that broad egalitarian principle is shared by all major political philosophers—liberal, socialist, communitarian and green. After all, who would wish to publicly declare themselves as being opposed to equality of opportunity?

Yet, in practice, obstacles to equality of opportunity abound. In the educational system, in health provision, in employment, in transport and in so many other fields, inequalities of access, affordability and outcome persist. Marginalised groups—whether identified by gender, ethnicity or location—do it tough. People with disabilities usually do it toughest of all. To be sure, individual acts of kindness and support abound, and public policies are often formally aimed at ameliorating the problems. No one is supposed to be a 'second-class citizen'. Yet, systemic features of the economy, society and political process commonly reproduce and intensify the problems of marginalisation and disadvantage.

That is why seeking social inclusion requires more than understanding and goodwill. It requires simultaneous consideration of broader political economic issues—how society is structured and how political economic power is used to serve some interests and deny others.

The influence of neoliberalism is particularly crucial in this regard. Neoliberal ideologies emphasise individual choice in the marketplace. Yet not all people are equally capable of effective choice or market participation. It follows that the increased influence of neoliberalism in public policy in recent years has become part of the problem. Arguably, so-called 'third-way' politics, posited as a modern alternative to a more long-standing tradition of social democracy, has similar features—emphasising the rhetoric of 'community' and 'big society' but withdrawing governmental support for those in need.

It is hard to imagine anyone better qualified to explore and analyse these issues than Peter Gibilisco, the author of this book. He has had to contend with a chronic physical disability that would render most people incapable of doing more than just surviving an extremely difficult day-to-day existence. Yet, Peter has pursued advanced education at two Melbourne campuses and travelled interstate and internationally to interview leading scholars at other universities. The award of a PhD for a thesis dealing with political theory and social disadvantage was the culmination of many years struggle and committed effort. Since completing his PhD, Peter has written numerous articles about his personal experience and politics of disability. Therein lies the origin of the ideas and analyses that he has compiled in this book. As you read on, you will see that it is written from 'the heart' as well as 'the head'—but only very, very slowly with the hands, as Peter's keyboard typing averages only about two words a minute. [Since the time of writing this has reduced dramatically.]

Blending the personal and the political is always hard work. And, of course, nothing is ever easy when coping with a severe personal disability. Readers of this book may well experience some of these tensions. Yet creating social change is not easy either. It requires critique of what currently is. It requires vision of what could and should be. It also requires ideas and strategies for getting from here to there. This book is part of that difficult journey. Please accept Peter's invitation to join him as he probes what it would take to bring to fruition the cherished Australian ambition of a 'fair go, mate'.

INTRODUCTION

The dominant political ideas strongly affect the opportunities that people experience. Some political ideologies promote competitive individualism, creating difficult conditions for people who, for whatever reason, experience relative disadvantage or marginalisation. Other political ideologies are more inclusive, collectivist or egalitarian. Even in that latter case, however, obstacles to full and equal citizenship may, in practice, persist.

During the last three decades a political and social shift has occurred, modifying the dominant political ideology. As a result, societies around the world are confronted by ongoing debate not only about the form and content of current ideologies, but which one is to predominate in any political context. With the collapse of communism and the advent of corporate globalisation, social experiences have been transformed. Neoliberalism has been the dominant political creed. As a mutation of classical liberalism, this rejigged ideology proclaims the absolute freedom of the individual person, and promotes more self-centred forms of political individualism. It flies in the face of more collectivist political economy actions that drove the earlier era called the 'golden age' of capitalism from the ground up.

Neoliberalism operates at the individual as well as the societal level. For neoliberals, it is 'all about me'. This is the idea that our world view has shifted from focusing on our task as minor players in a bigger, wider society, to the view that society, and pretty much everything else, is simply revolving around us and our needs.

Such profound social, political and attitudinal changes have together provoked people of social democratic inclination to rethink the policies and theories usually associated with the left. Social democratic politics is, thus, in a state of critical self-reflection. More precisely, in Australia, pragmatic social democracy faces profound challenges with, on the one hand, the emergence of neoliberal models of society and policy, and, on the other hand, the promotion of a 'third-way' approach to social and economic reform. This third-way approach seeks to combine the social justice concerns of pragmatic social democracy with the market-based economics of neoliberalism (Gibilisco, 2005a).

Challenges: personal and political

The current context, in which societies are confronted by on-going debate about which political priorities should dominate, can be viewed from many different perspectives. The global financial crisis and subsequent economic problems rippling around the world raise big questions about the effectiveness and sustainability of the neoliberal order. Recognition of growing inequalities between rich and poor intensifies the quest for greater social justice. Awareness of the particular problems faced by people with disabilities is another, sometimes overlooked, dimension. In Australia, for example, the national government has recently embraced a comprehensive disabilities insurance scheme, called the National Disability Insurance Scheme (NDIS). But how effectively can such reforms operate without changing the overarching politics of neoliberalism?

I want to think about this and ask the pertinent question: how should people with disabilities situate themselves in such a politically self-centred and individualistic society? Do such people simply follow this trend and live by a world view in which everything other than themselves is simply there to meet their needs?

Take my own case. I have a PhD, which I achieved late into the progression of my disability, Friedreich's ataxia. I was awarded this degree as a result of studies undertaken between the ages of 38 to 43. In the examiners' reports I received great commendation: I had achieved, it was said, a standard that was 'above average'. However, I am left to wonder. Where has all this motivation for self-improvement got me? Although my efforts are appreciated and, at times, I have received acclamations for my academic achievements, I am still on a full disability support pension.

If I am to take on the current world view, with its self-centred, political individualism, wouldn't I now view myself as a 'loser' because of my disability? I guess I would be sorely tempted to do so if I were to evaluate myself according to the tenets of neoliberalism. But that is just the point. I'm of the conviction that the advocates of such self-centred, political individualism have actually ended up 'losing the plot' by promoting a cruel and anti-humanist world view. Their 'survival of the fittest' dogmas have led us all astray about the value of the work that has to be done.

Let's probe deeper. Two problems in particular may be distinguished. First, the social rights of many of society's most vulnerable people are becoming politically extinct—their voices are simply not being heard above the din of self-interest. Second, the not-for-profit business philosophy that has been central to catering for the needs of vulnerable people is being compromised politically and ethically by the calculus that arises from an individualised way of thinking about political rights.

Let me run you through a brief example of what I perceive to be the emergent business philosophy of many not-for-profit service providers in the disability sector. The funding for most disability service providers, or at least a fair amount of them, is supplied by State government grants. The providers make bids for contracts to provide such services.

I can speak on this matter because, in terms of the stated rationale for such service provision, I am, as the person being served, the direct employer of the person through whom the agency receives their funding from the State government. Yet, for all the work involved in taking on this 'employer role', the government has never thought that I, as employer, should receive any funding to assist me in the exercise of my duties. What are my duties? They involve rostering, managing and overseeing payroll, WorkCover insurance, occupational health and safety, and arranging for flexible employment of employees. If I were to employ some academically qualified support workers to assist me with the professional duties associated with my employer status, I would not receive a 'brass razoo'.

On the other hand, disability service provision is mostly made up of providers that arise from not-for-profit agencies. The not-for-profit sector is supposedly made up of businesses that do not have the need to make a profit. That is, the not-for-profit sector does not have to worry about meeting shareholder demands—those who invest in a business and anticipate receiving a dividend from the company's profits.

The disability sector plays a large role in the not-for-profit sector. For example, many service providers are in receipt of government payments of $39.80 an hour, but the support workers they employ get about $20 an hour. If a service provider serves, say, 200 clients in one-on-one support, paying support workers about $20 an hour with each client being served for about 20 hours a week, by my calculations, that amounts to an annual income of approximately \$4 013 206. These figures are based on conservative estimates of the yearly income for these not-for-profit disability service providers.

The question here is whether there is a systemic injustice in the manner in which these funds are distributed. Are there a small number 'at the top' who live very well from a system generated by public funds provided to supply disability support to needy members of society? We recall the gratuitous attempts of financial institutions to justify the exorbitant remuneration of their senior executives. Is there a similar self-centred drive within the not-for-profit sector of service providers in the disability sector? Does this perhaps provide us with an important part of the structural injustices that lie behind the social dilemmas confronted by people with disabilities?

Studying social dilemmas is an essential purpose of social and political sciences. This can be seen when a collective act is in opposition to private interests. For example, a situation could be a short-term private (selfish) one or a long-term collective interest. This happens in such situations when either of the interests is given priority.

It was from within such social dilemmas, and by seeking to understand them, that my PhD thesis gained its major momentum. A central theme is that the blatant, individual self-interest promoted by neoliberalism is an acid that erodes the best attempts to publicly pursue justice in disability policy. Indeed, the conflicting ideologies of collectivism and neoliberalism actually seem to work together and derive momentum from each other. Proponents of the competing ideologies may tell us that their theories work, but, in practice, the factual outcomes pertaining to disability tell us something different.

A brief snapshot of my life

Let's get personal. Here's a brief statement of how I have had to struggle with a disability and consequent socioeconomic obstacles since a teenager. It was when I was 14 that I was diagnosed with Friedreich's ataxia. This is a progressive disease, causing impairment to the nerves, and so a failure of timely muscle reactions throughout my body. The messages sent from the brain via neurotransmitters are slower and weaker than they should be. In turn, muscular growth is hampered, giving rise to severe deformities, limitations and other problems. For example, I have had to deal with severe scoliosis and cardiomyopathy. By 23, I was reliant on a wheelchair, but now I'm simply too uncoordinated (unco) to make use of an electric one. As you may realise, the condition also leads to severely slurred speech, which by the time I was 40 meant my communication was also seriously impaired (Gibilisco, 2011g). Of late, my eyesight has been deteriorating, adding to the challenges that I already face.

When I was 18, my mother died of cancer. That put me well and truly on a downward emotional and physiological spiral. By 23, confined permanently to a wheelchair, I began studying for an Associate Diploma in Accountancy at Dandenong TAFE. How did that come about? I think a lot about that. I'm grateful for encouragement and perceptive advice from a close lady friend. Her straight talking and sensible advice lifted me out of a fantasy land of self-pity. Looking back, it was just what I needed. That inclusive and happy learning environment gave me inspiration to tackle life with vigour and it still serves as a reminder to me when, like anyone else, I develop the usual emotional itches that need scratching.

That was in 1984 (Gibilisco, 2006a; Gibilisco, 2008b).

Each of the steps I have made through my own higher education have deepened my desire to promote and harness the capabilities of people who, in diverse ways, are not snuffed out by disability. My qualifications include: the Dandenong TAFE Diploma; a Bachelor of Business; a Bachelor of Arts; and a Master of Arts—all from Monash University between the years of 1991 to 2000. Then I completed a Doctorate of Philosophy from the University of Melbourne (2000–2005).

The upshot of all that is my increased conviction that somehow we—all of us—need to find a way to view and support people with disabilities in proactive and caring ways, taking equal opportunity as a principle for a way of life that is flexible enough to assist diverse disablement in diverse ways. Rather than focusing on trying to combat the uncaring and judgemental stereotypes that arise from the biomedical model's view of sympathetic charity, we need simply to face up to people with severe disabilities *as people*. That is, we need a flexible and empathetic approach, aligned to an appreciation of the diverse social abilities, responsibilities and opportunities that become evident when people interact with each other as fellows, as equals.

My assertion is that our corporate responsibility increases in specific ways when those with severe disabilities take hold of the opportunities for professional development. Like any other student, a graduate with a disability is also on the verge of achieving a life's goal, which includes providing thankful service. The 'mutual obligation' has increased on all sides.

In 2007, I was presented with the Emerging Disability Leader Award. I also applied for many positions after graduating, after being 'doctored'. I am confident that I could have performed well in many of these positions, but I was unable to secure employment. The constraints that are assumed from a neoliberal economic perspective mean that even not-for-profit firms find it difficult to employ people like myself. I believe I know how to make a contribution that could improve or at least maintain viability of the services offered by such firms. But to this day my 'mutual obligation in public service' is channelled through board positions, which can never allow me the social inclusion that regular employment would provide.

In 2010, I sought to publish my thesis, my greatest achievement until then. But at that time no major mainstream Australian publishing house was eager to take on the risk of a book about disability. Why? Doesn't this only clarify at a deeper level the importance of such books and the subject matter they present to us? And so, after many negative and disheartening attempts with publishers, I finally went to a print-on-demand publisher based in Europe and the US, which, I believe, heavily overpriced my first book and therefore drastically reduced demand for it, and, hence, its influence.

In writing this current book I had no difficulty in arguing my case in political terms, which I've done, so I found myself happily plunging into the analysis of some of the major issues of the day, explaining the social exclusion of many people with disabilities—that is, people not unlike myself. The major difficulty I had was my far from adequate typing speed—only about two words a minute, and reducing all the time—which constantly created problems.

Confronting and analysing some of the political issues concerning people with disabilities has had its ups and downs. But the exercise has been productive and has reminded me of our potential in society as people with different—and, let it be said, in some cases better—abilities than those who are more fully able-bodied.

My recent and hopefully everlasting burst of encouragement arose, once again, through a mutually beneficial friendship. This has helped me get my life back on track when times appeared to be too difficult. Friendship—we can't do without it.

The structure of this book

The book develops a series of key themes: analysing neoliberalism; third-way social democracy; education; employment of people with severe physical disabilities; and service provision in the disability sector. Through these steps, the analysis moves from looking at broad social and political ideas and structures, considering the implications for people with disabilities, to looking at specific policy areas.

The different chapters of the book draw on material I have previously compiled for websites such as *On Line Opinion* (www.onlineopinion.com.au). The evidence, arguments and personal experience are put together here to illustrate the bigger picture. The book examines many socioeconomic and political dimensions of inequality, marginalisation and exclusion—particularly as they affect people with disabilities. It treats these problems as interdependent and cumulative. Hence, the great policy challenge to which I seek to contribute—trying to make a difference.

The general motivation for my book is the belief that we need a better understanding of how to create a genuinely inclusive society. It is not an easy journey, personally or politically, but it is critically important from the perspective of social justice.

Works Consulted

Gibilisco, P. (2005a), *The Political Economy of Disablement: A sociological analysis*, PhD Thesis, University of Melbourne.

Gibilisco, P. (2006a), 'A social study of success', *On Line Opinion*, February 14, 1–2, http://www.onlineopinion.com.au/view.asp?article=41 43.

Gibilisco, P. (2008b), 'Itches and Scratches—living with disability', *On Line Opinion*, March 19, 1–3, http://www.onlineopinion.com.au/view.asp?article=71 27.

Gibilisco, P. (2011g), *Politics, Disability and Social Inclusion: People with different abilities in the 21st Century*, VDM Verlag, Saarbrücken.

Wikipedia (2012), *Social Dilemma*, http://en.Wikipedia.org/wiki/Social_dilemma.

CHAPTER 1

Justice for People with Disabilities is Structured on Empowerment

According to Shakespeare (1998), there are approximately 50 million people with a disability in Europe.

...

and figures that reach 500 million worldwide (Shakespeare, 1998).

...

In the under resourced and 'developing' countries, there seems to be significantly more disabled people. However, prevalence of disability is highest in the wealthier 'disabled' societies (Shakespeare, 1998).

...

Due to the ageing population and the advancements in the medical field to prolong life, the number of people with disabilities will increase dramatically in the future. This will lead to far-ranging economic, political and social implications (Shakespeare, 1998).

What are the foundations for achieving a just society for people with disabilities? People with disabilities face a power struggle because they live in a world where they are oppressed by a society that sees ableism as the norm. This is a society that can, and does, place degrading hardships upon people with disabilities. These hardships then act as a barrier against people reaching their full potential. For example, this occurs when one or a group of society's so-called norms contribute to oppressive or discriminating acts on minority groups, including people with disabilities. Unfortunately, the disabled as a group lack the resources and often lack the drive and vocabulary to articulate their oppression. In effect, they are social outcasts.

Russell (2002) speaks of the alienation of people with disabilities within circles of social justice:

> It is disheartening, to say the least, when I can still pick up a book or read a call for unity to fight for social justice which omits or does not give equal weight to the disability social movement against oppression (Russell 2002: 1).

With these words, Russell identifies the disheartening production of politics that confronts people with disabilities. Most of these exclusionary factors are related both directly and indirectly to the 'biomedical model' and its preoccupation with ablest social norms. The functional restrictions faced by people with disabilities are imposed by human distortions of capabilities and opportunities, made worse by prejudice, discrimination, inaccessible environments and inadequate support.

In recent years, there has been some improvement for people with disabilities. This change has been brought about by the influence of a social model of disability that challenges the biomedical model, and by the, sometimes, pragmatic styling of disability research. The biomedical model of disability sees a disability as a diagnosable set of symptoms that either have to be alleviated or might entail the isolation of that person from wider society. The social model of disability views the physical or mental impairment as being a social construction, and believes the attitudes and prejudices about it are compounded by a lack of accessible and socially rewarding information, and by a lack of appropriate institutional arrangements (Gibilisco 2003a).

The consequences of the biomedical model

Disability historian Paul Longmore wisely concludes that the biomedical model (also more simply called the medical model) is most harmful because it presents disabled people with 'an impossible dilemma' (Russell 1998c:14).

The impossible dilemma to which Longmore refers is the biomedical model's systematic explanation of disability. Medicine cures and maintains people in our society. The biomedical model regards those people who are sick as requiring medicine and wanting to get well, including those with incurable conditions and those with disabilities who are classified as being sick. These people are, in effect, deviants from society's norm. Thus, the biomedical model creates a link between people with a disability and social deviance, which not only affects individual people with disabilities, but also influences health care and research, in turn supporting the continued dominance of professionally and medically controlled healthcare and welfare services for people with disabilities.

The experiences of disability are usually presented in the context of the medical implications, which are recognised to have, and viewed primarily as, a particular set of physical or intellectual dysfunctions. In this way, the myth comes to be shared by people with disabilities, believing that they require medical supervision as a permanent factor in their lives (Gibilisco 2003a).

The biomedical model posits that someone is disabled if the impairment has an effect on her or his life activities, not taking into account the infinite variety of social experiences and circumstances that can be found in daily activities. For example, a physical impairment that may have an adverse effect on a person's gait may be due to, or be exacerbated by, social and environmental factors, such as the design of transport systems that can also adversely affect mobility. Such factors are not reducible to medical factors, but, even so, the biomedical model judges people with disabilities to be deviant. Through such processes, the biomedical model is found to put highly contestable value judgements on human activities (Harrison 2000; Priestley 2001; Russell 1998c).

The biomedical model focuses on people's impairments rather than on their qualities or social circumstance. Traditionally, care for a person with disabilities was found within the extended family, and such care was usually provided by the female family members. The carer, in most circumstances, was described as a martyr or saint and the person with the disability was usually seen as their dependant, and under their family or professional control. It is disempowering for citizens (Harrison 2000:160–161).

The doctor–patient relationship highlights that many people with disabilities are treated as care recipients, as the doctor's interests are not always to act in the best interests of people with disabilities. Joe Harrison, an Australian disability activist and author, reported a personal example (Harrison 2000). The event took place during the costly but mundane medical procedure known as an electrocardiogram, where an individual is plugged into a machine that measures heartbeats. When Harrison experienced a major convulsion midway during the procedure, he mentioned that the doctor, rather than assisting him, chose to record the seizure. The doctor seemed to prefer improving his understanding on the pattern of Harrison's seizure than to assist him (Clear 2000). The biomedical model provides for a system where the needs of people with disabilities are not always a priority.

An example of this was given in June 1989, regarding a minister in Washington, DC, who has epilepsy. On an occasion after work and on the way home he had a seizure. From there he was taken directly to hospital by ambulance. When he woke, he got out of bed but was forced back into bed by three hospital security guards. At that time, of course, he protested and yelled, demanding to see a physician. But because of this, he was restrained and gagged. The guards had acted according to instructions from the medical staff, who believed patients with epilepsy were dangerous and needed to be forcefully restrained.

Clear (2000) and Priestley (2001) are among many who argue that people with disabilities are a socially excluded minority who are politically marginalised. For many of them, there is no known medical cure or treatment. To create a just society for all we must, therefore, alleviate and phase out any forms of social exclusion that hinder the fulfillment of so-called impaired people's lives and citizenship.

Fifteen years ago medical authorities responded conservatively to the need for a social model of disability, believing that there was not enough demand for it in their work. They said it was unsustainable, and that an understanding of the social model of disability is only needed by those with irredeemable disabilities. But, since then, the vast technological advances have created a whirlwind shift.

I personally am a 52-year-old who has a severe physical disability, Friedreich's ataxia, which at present cannot be cured. It is my belief, and the belief of many academics including Sen (1999), Priestley (2001) and Russell (2000a), that most capabilities and activities pertain to many norms that arise outside the biomedical model, but usually within the social model of people with disabilities. Harris has identified the biomedical model with all medical procedures. While there are clearly important medical procedures in the daily lives of most people with severe, incurable disabilities, that does not reduce the importance of their social opportunities. In other words, people with disabilities are not reducible to their medical constitution.

The consequences of the social model

The social model concerning people with disabilities started to become influential more than 20 years ago, both within the disabled persons' movement and as an influential driver in terms of social policy for people with disabilities. For example, when analysing mobility impairments, the social model asks why the environment is inaccessible and how it needs to be changed to accommodate people with disabilities. Brian Howe (2003), former deputy prime minister of Australia (1992–1995), understands the social model as taking:

> A social approach towards people with disabilities that emphasises the capacity of people to relate to others, and to develop their capacities in response to their attitudes to society, as well as societal attitudes towards them. The development of people with disabilities is largely influenced by societal expectations. This is obvious if you think of the changes that have taken place in recent decades (Howe 2003).

Nobody can deny the sincere empathy and compassion of the collective public contribution of social security benefits to people with disabilities. However, the social model is developed partly to move beyond this system. Like its namesake, the social model is a strand of social science, prompting us to continually consider the means required to encourage satisfying ends. But this is not to deny the need for adequate social security for people with disabilities; rather it is to argue the contrary. The social model recognises that people with disabilities face many barriers to leading a fulfilling social, cultural and economic life. That is, health is a social construction and experience, not purely constructed within the bio-medical science. As with poverty, in many cases the solutions are more than merely economic, although economic barriers can be substantial. Living at levels of subsistence is an unfortunate reality for many people with disabilities, which can rule out many of the activities that lift the spirit and encourage self-esteem (Gibilisco 2003a).

The social model has raised confusion in some recent debates about its supposed limitations. Critics believe it creates a false approach to impairment in terms of pain, illness, depression, fatigue, and so on. When disabilities arise from the way society treats physically impaired people there are two truths, which are not necessarily contradictory: the disability would be less if the social barriers did not exist; the disability would also be less if there was no impairment (Stretton 2003). Any medical reduction of the impairment is good. Any reduction of the social barriers is good, too!

While critics of the biomedical model accuse it of diverting attention away from the social barriers, and encouraging the belief that the individual impairment is the main or only cause of the disability, some critics of the social model claim that it exaggerates some impaired people's capacity for social and economic activity, arguing that the medical barriers are such that the social barriers do not add much to the sufferers' deficiency. Between those views it is possible to disagree about the practical possibilities of social reform (Stretton 2003). But none of these problems of judgement, which can differ from case to case, should discredit the social model, or justify a belief in the biomedical model alone.

In his introduction to the book *Promises Promises*, Clear (2000) discusses the social approach to disability that sees impairment as not being necessarily tragic. Impairment can be seen as a function of human diversity, but it can bring systematic discrimination and exclusion from mainstream society. Clear (2000) argues that the trouble is in the disabling society. The lives of people labelled as impaired or disabled should have the same value as people who live without those labels. Impairment may cause pain and discomfort, but the real disability arises from a sociocultural system that does not recognise everyone's right to equal treatment. People with disabilities face many barriers, including attitudinal, economic, architectural, and sensory. There may also be an over-dependence on professionals. Often, there is inadequate support to overcome these barriers. Perhaps the solution lies in providing assistance to remove these barriers by giving self-advocacy, system advocacy, and control to the disabled person.

The biomedical model has traditionally placed many stereotypes, stigmas and disutilities upon me and many other people with disabilities. For example, I have been pitied, conveniently verbally misunderstood, looked down on for my so-called or supposed abnormal structure and characteristics, and characterised as a loser. Over the years, I have come to understand most people's roles in reinforcing and amplifying the barriers to social inclusion are due to their lack of accessible information about disability. If, according to the biomedical model, such problems are a reflection of my severe disability, the question arises, which model best explains my successful completion of a PhD?

Dignity of risk should be a disability right

There is a concept called 'dignity of risk'. This refers the right of everyone to pursue activities that have a level of risk, for example, going swimming or surfing. However, the risk can be managed by, in this case, checking the conditions before going, and going with a friend. So does this mean that a service provider or carer of someone with a disability has to balance the risk to the disabled person and the right of that person to pursue happiness for them? People with disabilities are usually in the best position to instruct their own support services. Dignity of risk should mean that support services encourage the disabled to make their own informed choices.

Stereotyping and discriminatory attitudes can make it even more difficult for a person with disabilities to be a 'normal person'. It follows that the disabled person should decide for him or herself what their own 'dignity of risk' level is. Recognition of this need will facilitate a better relationship between the support workers and the disabled.

The danger is that the principle dignity of risk is something that can be over-ridden—and the disabled persons' support turned into a legal tug of war. Sometimes people with a disability are prevented from making certain decisions or participating in activities because other people judge these to be too risky. How risk is perceived is unique to us as individuals and management of risk should be tailored to a person's individual circumstances.

Section 69 of the Victorian
Equal Opportunity Act 1995

Are the above principles legally enforced so as to ensure the upholding of disability rights? Consider Section 69 of the Victorian *Equal Opportunity Act 1995*:

> A person may discriminate if the discrimination is necessary to provision of an Act, other than the Equal Opportunity comply with, or is authorised by, an Act (RNDS, 2012).

In other words, other legislation can override laws against discrimination and disregard dignity of risk for the disabled.

What are these 'rights' that can be overridden by other legislation? Is there to be real justice—or the rhetoric of concern? The exemption clause, Section 69 of the Victorian *Equal Opportunity Act*, appears to place a second-class status upon people with disabilities.

For example, in 2002, I contacted the Equal Opportunities Department about a dispute I was having with the Royal District Nursing Service. This issue was directly related to Occupational Health and Safety laws (RNDS, 2012). Upon contacting the Equal Opportunities Department, however, I was confronted with Section 69 of the Victorian *Equal Opportunities Act*. So, I was making my appeal in terms of dignity of risk—while my dignity could be overridden by an appeal to Section 69.

The administrators of the Victorian *Equal Opportunity Act* will be hard-pressed to ensure that the human rights of people with disabilities will be fully respected.

An inclusive society for people with disabilities

The post-World War II period developed a concept of the useful human, usually male with no disabilities, which contributed to the development of stigmas and disutilities concerning people with disabilities (Johnson 2002). Welfare in the post-World War II period assisted in leaving behind some of the stereotypes concerning people with disabilities.

Priestley (2001) acknowledges that this helped in the creation of the 'International Year of the Disabled Person' in 1981, and argues that the politics of people with disabilities has helped to create a concentrated effort to develop new policies to increase social inclusiveness.

It can be argued that globalisation has created opportunities for people with disabilities by encouraging a form of social inclusion. At the forefront, at least in theory, are the social-policy mechanisms of the third-way (Stretton 2003). The third-way points to the failings of traditional social democracy and the welfare state for the social exclusion of people with disabilities. The third-way needs to reflect on the criticisms and recommendations of political bodies to advance all social inclusion, and to offer people with disabilities new and exciting methods to help build barriers against social exclusion. Global economic competition can assist and act as a driving force in the development of technology for people with disabilities, including in the work environment. Modernisation in all walks of life—including in welfare, education, public consultation, technology, and so on—driven by government policies, businesses, and the pressures of geographical and demographic changes have created new prospects for people with disabilities.

The paradox pertaining to the third-way and pragmatic social democracy rests in the contradictory values of theory and practice. In theory, the third-way's grand plan for people with disabilities is structured according to the social model of disability, as highlighted in the Victorian ALP's State Disability Plan, which reflects many of the current third-way principles of social inclusiveness for people with disabilities. Key elements of this plan include:

- a new approach to disability that is based on fundamental principles of human rights and social justice ('The Way Forward')

- the principle of dignity and self-determination (choice), i.e. respecting and valuing the knowledge, abilities and experiences that people with a disability possess, supporting them to make choices about their lives, and enabling each person to live the life they want to live ('Guiding principles')

- disability supports to focus on supporting people with a disability in flexible ways, based on their individual needs, so that each person can live the lifestyle that they want to lead ('The New Approach')

- a commitment to monitoring its progress and evaluating the outcomes of the priority strategies that it puts into place, ensuring that real progress is made towards achieving the Government's vision in the next 10 years ('Next steps') (Department of Human Services 2002a).

The State Disability Plan was introduced in 2002 by the Victorian Labor government, under reforms to the disability services sector. In its language, the State Disability Plan draws on the theoretical claims of third-way social democracy, in particular the coexistence of rights and responsibilities. This poses the controversial and paradoxical idea of mutual obligation for people with disabilities.

The emphasis on support services in the personal care of people with disabilities has allowed the government, in practice, to heighten the confusion about government policies that deal with the support services for people with disabilities. An example is where my responsibilities to life are measured by my dedication and achievement in the field of academia, which is excellent given my impairments. However, I am still not able to receive the required and adequate care and support, even under the State Disability Plan. The State Disability Plan's flexible social democratic theory is held back from becoming practice because of the Victorian ALP's reliance on third-way policies that are dependent on economic stylings of neoliberalism. In practice, I receive diminished rights even though I have exceeded in my responsibilities[1].

Russell (2001a) argues that the social exclusion of people with disabilities is promoted by the third-way's practical pursuit of neoliberal economic policies. As Russell (2000a) has stated:

> [I]t is safe to say that any full solution to the unemployment predicament of disabled persons under [the third-way or neo-liberalism] cannot depend on liberal civil rights anti-discrimination measures and the random integration of disabled people into the economy that civil rights promise (but so far have not delivered) (Russell 2000a:5).

Russell (2000a) asks: what role is to be played by the new

---

[1] I finally received a more adequate personal care package from Disability Services from June 2007.

economy in developing a vision of a just society? In particular, is the new economy to support market-driven profits and models of production that exclude segments of the population, or should the role of the new economy be to help sustain social bonds that help to create a socially inclusive society for all, including people with disabilities? The answer must be to support putting people before profits (Russell 2001a; see also: Howe 2003; Stilwell 2002; Stretton 2003).

Insights into my life

Russell (2003b) refers to the unnecessary hardships that many people with disabilities experience as follows:

> Physical, social, political, economic, and cultural barriers keep millions of disabled children and adults throughout the world excluded from fundamental citizenship (Russell, 2003b).

They often fall short of attaining or enjoying any human rights and remain absent from social and productive activities. Disabled persons face barriers to accessible education, employment, health care, transportation, public facilities and housing. Participation in social and political groups is limited or denied them. They are cut off from affectionate relationships and even denied the right to move. Possibilities that allow most persons to develop a desired lifestyle are out of reach due to the construction of societies in which they live (Russell 2003b:1).

Personally, the gradual and insistent progress of my disease, Friedreich's ataxia, has created a system of social exclusion. Of course, there have been many enriching and fulfilling occasions that I have shared with beautiful people. However, the horrible and despicable times certainly have occurred much more often than the good. Some individuals, out of frustration and disbelief at seeing what I have to put up with, ask me, 'What is the point of your carrying on with this existence?' I reply in a similar way to most people, 'I proceed in the hope that maybe one day there will be a reversal of fortune, and I will be able to share in more good times.' Further, I am motivated by the belief that my work can contribute to changing this situation generally for people with disabilities (Gibilisco 2005:1).

In being motivated by the hope for better times, I have attempted and succeeded in the pursuit and achievement at most levels of higher education (Gibilisco 2003b:9; Gibilisco 2006a). I have struggled to achieve, in a world that does not give much, or the right forms of, acknowledgement to people with disabilities and in many instances openly, and in more hidden ways, discriminates. The social model would create the social environment that allows many people with disabilities to attempt and possibly achieve their goals, with less hindrance. Ideally, the social model of disability could liberate most people with disabilities from human-made social, economic, political, cultural and environmental oppression (Gibilisco 2005:1).

Many people with disabilities carry the burdensome and discriminatory tags that are created by the biomedical model, as most of these people also suffer with the ever-challenging problem of overcoming or sustaining a medical impairment. The biomedical model can, however, view the display of such courage as irrelevant. The goal of the biomedical model is to cure and assist medical disabilities, not to find solutions to the economic, environmental, political, social, and cultural problems that have become the featured domains of the social model. As Russell (2003b) states:

All too often the medical model persists and ignorance of the social model of disablement dominates. The social model emphasizes that institutions—the political, economic, social, cultural organization of society— impose 'disability' upon those who have impairments by segregating and excluding them from the rights others enjoy (Russell 2003b:1).

The orthodoxies of the biomedical model have persistently helped to impose stigmas and disutilities upon people with disabilities (Gibilisco 2001:17). The medical model infers that people with disabilities may never equate to any form of acceptable social normalcy without a complete cure. This leaves those who cannot be cured carrying the unpopular burden of being socially defiant of normalcy, and, therefore, excluded. This leads to the social, economic, political and cultural marginalisation of many people with disabilities.

As I have said earlier, today I am 52 years old and hold a PhD, which is a very high honour for even the most able-bodied. There is some recognition, but not the due recognition for attaining such an achievement, against all odds. Or, as Russell (2002) puts it:

> [D]isability theorists have posed that under capitalism impairment is socialized as a specific form of oppression—disability. The defining feature of capitalism, commodity relations, has been a primary force behind the economic impoverishment of impaired persons. The material relation is primary and the ideology of superiority/inferiority serves the function of maintenance and perpetuation of this social relation (Russell 2002:4).

The social and economic achievement of living independently for the past 21 years on its own contradicts the implications of a severe disability according to the orthodoxies of the biomedical model. However, such an achievement is mundane when we take into consideration my success in academia. Through my faith, dedication and understanding of the social implications of attending university with a severe disability, I have achieved this, even though some of my physical abilities are severely reduced from those of society's so-called norms (Gibilisco 2006a).

Despite the limits of the biomedical model, most medically diagnosed impairments will require continued medical support, and medical doctors, medicines and the biomedical models will continue to have a role to play in the lives of many people with disabilities. At the same time, however, the unjust stigmas and disutilities that concern people with disabilities have been aided and abetted by the development of the biomedical model (Gibilisco 2005:2).

I believe the following example highlights the paradox that may prevail when we have too much of one model and not enough of the other. In 1987, a friend of mine with Friedreich's ataxia, the same disease I have, was to be married to the guy of her dreams, an able-bodied individual. However, as she signed the register, she got too excited, had a heart attack and died. The wedding was a beautiful moment, and the embodiment of the social model, in particular, allowing for the full participation of all people in a social activity. In hindsight, however, what should have been done medically to prevent the heart attack, remains the domain of the biomedical model. In other words, it is the interaction of the medical and social models that is important. The challenge of the present period is the dominance of the biomedical model (Gibilisco 2005:2).

The goal of the social model is to encourage mechanisms that make society more justly inclusive of people with disabilities. Most of my life with the disability, and especially over the past 18 years, my exposure to the biomedical model of disability has been very limited. It is because of time and mobility limits, as I wished to achieve my goals in a similar time to that of most able-bodied people who have previously achieved such goals. For example, on many occasions, I have continually postponed medical doctors' appointments, through the lack of funding or because of being too busy to attend, to the stage that I ended up not going at all (Gibilisco 2005:2).

My life, to a large degree, has been structured in accordance with the social model of people with disabilities. I felt no reason to appreciate or place any belief in the theories of the biomedical model that would view me as inferior to society's norm. Denial of this model has allowed me to concentrate on my studies and make goals for myself, like many others in society (Gibilisco 2005:2). However, since graduating with my PhD, I have been able to get out more, and experience first-hand the stereotypes, stigmas and disutilities that oppress people with severe physical disabilities, including that of having severely slurred speech. I have outlined some of

these oppressive behaviours in greater detail in other chapters.

Stretton (2003) argues for the need to seek the correct balance between the social and biomedical models of disability, which is acknowledged to be a major contributor to a happy and justified life. In all aspects of life it is an essential undertaking to try and maintain the correct balance between the two models of disability as a driving factor for success and happiness in all of life's pursuits. The correct balance will assist people with disabilities make necessary strategic choices, about how and what to prioritise in life.

But to ensure this, people with disabilities need to move beyond individual aspirations to harness the collective virtues of social empowerment, which will also need the adequate collective assistance of the state. Such action may ultimately lead to the creation of a just society for people with disabilities.

Love, sex, disability and stereotypes

Why is it so not normal to see the word 'disability' in this context? Such questions have been pondered over time, but most answers pertain to social norms, not the reality of humanity. Disability should not be unfairly subjected to stereotypes.

Is beauty truly in the eye of the beholder? Rather, beauty is in the mind of the beholder; acknowledging that beauty is not a quality that is understood as inherent. In real terms, beauty is reliant on interpretation, which may be beheld in either objective or subjective terms. While true meaningful love can inadequately be subjective, in reality, true and meaningful love is generally objective.

OK, generally what is believed to be beautiful and sexy can be subjective according to culture, personality and appearance. On the other hand, levels of objectivity are not without attainment in love, relationships, sexiness and beauty. Such objectivity within inter-ability relationships is happening today and will vastly increase in the future.

I had conducted some research on inter-ability relationships between those depicted as being extremely disabled. The results were interesting and heart warming, to say the least. One of my most recent research endeavours was to tour the website of both Megan (able bodied) and Barton (severe cerebral palsy) (Cutter and Cutter, 2014), focusing on their marriage and love life. They also shared a passion to communicate with the written word. Their ability to love and laugh together was founded on the mutual passion for writing. Barton and Megan Cutter went on to publish a book titled *Ink in the Wheel: Stories to Make Love Roll.*

Barton and Megan Cutter's book inspires me on so many levels. It brings us to a point of reflection about what is the true meaning of life.

The key to me seems to lie in a person's objectivity towards what matters in life, one must look to an equitable compromise in times of disagreement. But is this not a major contributing factor within many forms of true love? Love is a powerful force that has greedy humans persisting with negative stereotypes to make their own inadequacies feel better. For example, the truly pathetic stereotypes of the inadequate few when they talk about a person with a severe disability who drools—such heartless stereotypes that degrade another human's abilities.

Such unjust and demeaning stereotypes play a major role

with how one depicts themselves in society. Since I was diagnosed with Friedreich's ataxia, a severely progressive disability, 38 years ago, I have been no stranger to inter-ability relationships, but finding the right person to be able to handle me and my disability has been difficult. So have been the demeaning and deplorable stereotypes held by many in society that I have encountered. Such attitudes have made it difficult for me to create, develop and sustain such relationships.

I do not know or understand the reasons why I enjoy the chance or the fulfilment of making love. I guess it's because I am human. For example, this is the only human form of pleasure I am still capable of performing. While, my ability to perform may be dwindling on a level of consciousness, my ability to love has increased. And for the life of me I don't see why I also have to combat the utterly ridiculous stereotypes of others. Despite their thinking and coherent logical responses, I do not have a cognitive disability, but like many stereotypes this is, to some degree, an inescapable societal reality, but not a fact. It is only the fulfilment of social misguidance.

Social misguidance is still alive and feeds off uneducated degrading humour that disrespects different cultures, and only further enforces negative stereotypes. For me, it is so socially and culturally degrading to have such negative uneducated sayings (as seen earlier in this subchapter) carry such weight in the depiction of social norms.

Disability must be treated on an individual basis. After all, disability is much more than a political, individual scientific tool that is full of rhetoric.

A just society for people with disabilities

I suppose I am something of an agitator for the rights of the severely disabled. Despite my severe impediment, some years back I conducted some interviews—this during the jet-setting phase of my student life from my motorised wheelchair—and I was privileged to interview some of Australia's top political economic thinkers.

I found myself thinking about what these fellows said to me back then when they graciously accepted my requests for an interview, when I was fired up with all the energy of a bright young PhD candidate (I was actually just 38 at the time).

What I give here are some of my thoughts as to why they should be listened to by Australians (and any others) who are seeking to promote a just and equitable economy for all.

First, Frank Stilwell, Professor of Political Economy at the University of Sydney. Stilwell is a well-known critic of conventional economics and an advocate of alternative economic strategies that prioritise social justice and economic sustainability (Department of Political Economy, 2012). He talked openly and honestly with me about his political visions and aspirations for a just society. He opened the batting with this straight drive:

> [H]aving a just society is the ultimate goal in politics. If I can make play on words, we need a just society not just a society. We need a society that is cohesive, that is equitable and involves cooperative activity as well as healthy competition among its members (Department of Political Economy, 2012).

Of course, there are hurdles inhibiting the achievement of this goal. (Actually, I know a lot about obstacles. You can't avoid them from a wheelchair. And I have had to overcome some serious physical and psychological ones as well, but not only my own.) Stilwell believes that, in the struggle to achieve a just society, there are four major hurdles to be overcome:

1. the ecology problem—the ability to live in harmony with nature

2. the problem of peace—if we cannot live in peace with each other, fine tuning the economy is pointless

3. the need for social cohesion—understanding that it is the political and social processes by which we live together cooperatively and reign over economic inequality

4. the problem of the need for security and stability— most significantly that the unemployed must have a right to work. There is a need to create the capacity to allow all people from all walks of life to achieve economic security and stability. For example, we must create a context in which people with disabilities are able to work and/or be educated at university.

This will help to further promote the social inclusion of people with disabilities.

Stilwell defines himself in the words of Antonio Gramsci (1891–1937), believing he is 'a pessimist of the intellect but an optimist of the will'. Despite the prevalence of awful acts in the world today, Stilwell remains optimistic—he inspires me—and he is an ardent believer in the values mentioned above, and that they will ultimately become part of our social norms and produce a just society, possibly at some stage during the 21st century, maybe not tomorrow, or the next day, but maybe in 40 or 50 years' time. Stilwell believes that we will have to come to terms with our common humanity, with our common need for ecological sustainability, along with our need for peace and social cohesion. In creating a new social order, as Niccolo Machiavelli (1469–1527), one of history's greatest political minds, argues, we can learn from our past actions and mistakes to create a better future. There is a need to reconcile with our political past, not just dismiss it as a failure.

I also interviewed Professor Michael Pusey, Professor of Sociology at the University of New South Wales. I recall how he explained to me what he believed to be the fundamentals of a just society—those that can be fostered by a mixed economy. It is one in which all the features of the mixed economic and social approach contribute to the support of families and civil society. For such an approach to work effectively, both public and private sectors must work together to provide a just, peaceful and cohesive society. Pusey believes the key to a just society is found in the synergy of the sectors. Thus, strong private and public sectors equate with a vibrant economy, with a strong and active social presence, combined with a cohesive civil society.

My third political economic thinker of note is the historian Professor Stuart Macintyre. He argues that one must make use of the social aspects of social justice to facilitate egalitarian means and ends in society. He also argues that there should be more of a material economic acceptance of workers within organisations that provide services to people with disabilities. Since many of these services cannot be standardised, the human touch is always an essential component. That is something upon which I continue to reflect.

Then there is Professor Hugh Stretton, a political analyst and economist from whom I have learnt so much. His work has kept me pursuing this project of social justice, particularly in those long days when I had to type at just two words a minute to get my thesis into shape. Forgive me if I am a little misty eyed as I write this.

Stretton states:

> [E]verything from good parenting and child care through elaborate education and public and private research and development to an energetic and friendly culture help to contribute to [society]. Thus parents, teachers, researchers, writers and artists, and business and public managers all contribute to [society]. But so do the energies, skills and friendly and cooperative capacities of the whole population (Gibilisco, 2000).

This is the argument that is obvious to me—that there is a need to recognise any contribution to the work of society by any of its members, irrespective of the financial–reward dimensions of such work. For example, providing services to people with disabilities may not contribute much to economic growth, but it is fundamental to a just society. It provides a foundation for recognising and valuing our common humanity.

So there it is. I leave these reminiscences to speak for themselves. Thanks to Frank, Michael, Stuart and Hugh. I hope your work continues to inspire students like it has inspired me.

Action in Australian disability rights

In May 2011, a few thousand people attended a London rally to protest against cuts in government spending for services to people with disabilities. Here we witness people with disabilities demonstrating their political power. The mood is captured in an article published before the rally, which explains why the government's actions had actually triggered this protest: the government is replacing the 'Incapacity Benefit' with an 'Employment and Support Allowance' (ESA), and has contracted a private company, Atos Healthcare, to carry out tests on all those who are claiming it to assess whether they are capable of working. Atos uses computer-based tests, which are carried out by health workers, many of whom are not qualified doctors, and who are only allowed a short time to reach decisions in what are often complex cases.

The protest, in Britain, was a part of a National Week of Action against Atos Origin organised by disability activists, and more than 50 disability groups being politically proactive against such reforms. Many disabled activists were and are unable to get to demonstrations such as these, or fear to do so as it might prejudice their capability in work assessments, and, instead, take part in online protests as part of the 'Armchair Army'.

So, is such a demonstration of such obvious political anger possible in Australia? I think it is improbable. Even though there was a call for such action in the last South Australian State election, the election of a Dignity for Disability Rights candidate to the legislative assembly perhaps shows a greater depth of public sensitivity to those cared for, and their carers and support workers. That is not to say that we are perfect simply because we don't have to face the draconian testing of the Conservative Liberal Democratic Coalition government in the United Kingdom.

Here I think the question is about keeping up the political pressure to enhance disability rights in Australia. Why does this prove to be so difficult? A clear example of what we are up against was visible in 2007 when I was a Senate candidate for the Carers' Alliance. In that capacity I happily arranged to attend a few disability rallies, but when only a handful of people turned up it becomes hard to make any media impact and, therefore, all the more difficult to bring political pressure to bear on other candidates and on the other parties' agendas.

Yet, we have seen some 'disability awareness' in a cogent political sense, with Kelly Vincent taking her seat in the South Australian legislative assembly. Kelly is the first person using a wheelchair to be elected to the South Australian parliament, and also the first Australian parliamentarian elected on a disability platform. The opportunity is there for disability rights activists to generate greater awareness and, thus, for Australian society to place greater value upon changes that will enhance the rights of people with disabilities. There is a need for much more political acceptance and action from the major parties, which will then make it feasible for more candidates, like Kelly, to take on public political roles around the country. This will also allow the voice of the disabled to be heard where it needs to be heard.

One doesn't have to be a genius or mentally gifted to realise that a significant growth in political awareness would result if those people directly related to the issues of disability would stick together and find ways, including voting, to have their voice heard in Australian political life. A federal, state, or local party that insists on upholding the full political dignity of people with disabilities—which has to include encouraging their active political participation—will in time gather support from the disabled community, but the task is also to see that such changes to our view of political participation must be of benefit to everyone.

Political power today becomes decentralised when it is dominated by a view that gives in to arguments about the budget bottom line. That has proved a sure way to avoid the most urgent social justice needs. Lobby groups in Victoria, which are active in backing and promoting such services, in particular for people with disabilities, their carers and support workers, for instance, are quite poor, to the point of being almost irrelevant. Nevertheless there is a vital job here to politically assist, promote and empower such groups. Victorians who are directly and indirectly involved with disability should take time to ponder the question about our own political responsibility: how can we best use the abilities of the many people and groups involved in disability to make ourselves more visible and to convince our neighbours of the great relevance of our cause?

The political progress of disability rights in Australia is indeed out of whack with, and fails most measures of, social justice. We live in a society where our most vulnerable are forced to carry the load of this imbalance. It is viewed as an individual's burden rather than a shared responsibility. This in itself brings with it new forms of social ignorance, where many people not only forget but encourage an ethos of social impoverishment. Let it be said that this may also indirectly be the result of how our politicians and their parties have set their agendas to argue about bottom-line management.

This is an ongoing political fight for every one of us, not just for people with disabilities. There should not be the constant battle about a politically enforced social-justice compromise that holds us all back.

In the UK they are seen to be more politically proactive concerning the social policy for people with disabilities. By believing and politically acting out such beliefs, it's possible, to have a society that is not reliant on the exploitation of others, but which stipulates the equality of all human beings. Australia has some way to go before we can say we have got to the point where those who indirectly and directly benefit and make use of such services are also making a political difference for the entire country.

Works Consulted

Clear, M. (2000), 'Introduction', *Promises Promises*, Clear, M. (ed), The Federation Press, Annandale, xiii–xvi.

Cutter, B. & Cutter, M. (2014), 'Success Comes Through Motivation and Perseverance: Barton and Megan Cutter Purchase MV-1 Accessible Vehicle', *Love Rolls On*. Posted on January 5, http://www.loverollson.com/blog/.

Department of Human Services (2012c), Supporting decision making: A guide to supporting people with a disability to make their own decisions. Disability Services: Department of Human Services, available from http://www.dhs.vic.gov.au/__data/assets/pdf_file/0011/690680/dsd_cis_supporting_decision_making_0212.pdf.

Department of Political Economy (2012), Professor Frank Stilwell. University of Sydney, available from http://sydney.edu.au/arts/political_economy/staff/academic_staff/frank_stilwell.shtml.

Department of Work and Pensions (2011), Employment and Support Allowance: Department of Work and Pensions, available from http://www.dwp.gov.uk/employment-and-support/.

Gibilisco, P. (2000), 'Hugh Stretton and His Social Theory', *Journal of Economic and Social Policy*: Vol. 5: Iss. 1, Article 5, available from http://epubs.scu.edu.au/jesp/vol5/iss1/5.

Gibilisco, P. (2001), 'Student profile', From Mayhem to Masters: tips and information for managing uni when you have a disability, University of Melbourne Disability Liaison Unit, Melbourne, 17.

Gibilisco, P. (2003a), 'A Just Society: Inclusive of people with disabilities', *Journal of Australian Political Economy*, Number 52:128–142, http://www.jape.org/Jape52_11_Gibilisco.pdf.

Gibilisco, P. (2003b), 'A Pragmatic Social Democrat: An Interview with Hugh Stretton', *Journal of Australian Political Economy*, Volume 1, Number 51, 132–142.

Gibilisco, P. (2003c), 'A Study in Success', *Campus Review: your sector your newspaper*, Volume 13, Number 25, July 2nd–8th, 9.

Gibilisco, P. (2005b), 'Treating disabled as 'patients' leads to stigmas and discrimination', *On Line Opinion* , March 7, 1–2, http://www.onlineopinion.com.au/view.asp?article=3103.

Gibilisco, P. (2006a), 'A social study of success', *On Line Opinion*, February 14, 1–2; http://www.onlineopinion.com.au/view.asp?article=4143.

Gibilisco, P. (2011a), 'Action in Australian Disability Rights', *On Line Opinion*, June 14, 1, http://www.onlineopinion.com.au/view.asp?article=12173.

Gibilisco, P. (2011c), 'Dignity of Risk should be a disability right', *On Line Opinion*, March 29, 1–2, http://www.onlineopinion.com.au/view.asp?article=11819.

Gibilisco, P. (2011i), 'Three Encounters', *On Line Opinion* ,
    July 12, 1–2,
    http://www.onlineopinion.com.au/view.asp?article=12
    308.

Harris, J. (2000), 'Is there a coherent social conception of
    disability?', *Journal of Medical Ethics*, Volume 26, Is-
    sue 2, 95–105.

Harrison, J. (2000), 'Models of care and social perceptions of
    disability', *Promises Promises*, Clear, M (ed), The
    Federation Press, Annandale, 159–169.

Howe, B. (2003), Interview with Peter Gibilisco, unpub-
    lished.

Johnson, C. (2002), Interview with Peter Gibilisco, unpub-
    lished.

Priestley, M. (2001), 'Introduction: the global context of dis-
    ability', *Disability and the Life course: global Per-
    spectives*, Priestley, M. (ed), Cambridge University
    Press, Cambridge, 3–14.

Pusey, M (2002), Interview with Peter Gibilisco, unpublished.

RNDS (2012), Royal District Nursing Service. Available from http://www.rdns.com.au/p.

Russell, M. (1998b), *Beyond Ramps: Disability at the End of the Social Contract*, Common Courage Press, Monroe—Maine.

Russell, M. (2000a), 'The Political Economy of Disablement', *Dollars and Sense*, September, 1–7, http://www.disweb.org/marta/ped.html.

Russell, M. (2000b), 'Why not capitalism', Z net: Daily commentaries, http://www.zmag.org/ZSustainers/ZDaily/2000-05/20russell.htm.

Russell, M. (2002), 'The Social Movement Left Out', Z net: Daily commentaries, 1–5. http://www.zmag.org/sustainers/content/2002-08/31russell.cfm.

Russell, M. (2003), 'Nothing About Us Without Us: Human Rights and Disability', Z net Daily Commentaries, 1–4, http://www.zmag.org/sustainers/content/2003-07/25russell.cfm.

Sen, A. (1999), *Development as Freedom*, Anchor Books, New York.

Shakespeare, T. (1998), *The Disability Reader: Social Science Perspectives*. Cassell Publishing.

Stilwell, F. (2002), Interview with Peter Gibilisco, unpublished.

Stretton, H. (2003), Interview with Peter Gibilisco, unpublished.

CHAPTER 2

Neoliberalism and Its Impact on People with Disabilities

> The aim of neoliberalism is to put into question all col-
> lective structures capable of obstructing the logic of
> the pure market. In particular, we situate our analysis
> within the rise of increased global economic competi-
> tion and neo-liberal policies in which the government
> seeks to retain legitimacy by instituting reforms to re-
> duce governmental expenditures on social services
> and, if possible, to privatize them (Hursh, 2003:6).

Neoliberalism is a political economic theory and practice that
emerged in the 1960s, and has increased in prominence at the
policy level since the 1980s. The neoliberal approach rejects
social democratic doctrines. Neoliberalism focuses politically
on the establishment of a stable medium of exchange, the reduction of localised rules, regulations and barriers to com-
merce, and the privatisation of state-run enterprises.

This contemporary, dominant, economic ideology of most
western countries is referred to as neoliberalism because it is

a modern version of the classical liberalism that initially arose in the 18th century. Moreover, neoliberalism claims to be a political system designed to highlight both the political limitations of the market economy in the nation-state, and the economic efficiency and effectiveness of the market economy when it is freed to operate on a global scale.

Prominent authorities cited in the neoliberal argument are Adam Smith, who is usually misrepresented, and Milton Friedman, the major economic promoter of free market economics. Smith is believed to be the theoretical founder of neoliberal economics, while Friedman is known as the creator of monetarism. Neoliberals regard Smith as their prophet because they believe he demonstrated how self-interest creates the best possible social order resulting in the best possible outcomes for all, including using society's resources to their fullest potential.

Classical liberal economics was developed by Adam Smith, at the beginning of the industrial revolution. Smith argued that government intervention disrupted the natural order of society. According to Smith, the natural order of society can be defined as a society left to its own devices. Smith based his economic beliefs on the argument that most economic self-interest is altruistic. This can be noted in his famous quote from *The Wealth of Nations*:

> 'It is not from the benevolence of the butcher, the brewer, or the baker, that we expect our dinner, but from their regard to their own interest.' (Smith, 1976 [1776]: book 1, chapter I, 18)

Can individual self-interest be altruistic? Of course, but the chances of it being plainly selfish and greedy are greater. As can be witnessed today by the problematic growth in the economic divide between rich and poor that is encountered in everyday life by those in general society.

According to Smith, this classical liberal system would provide for an economic infrastructure that could not only provide economic benefits, but also help promote a proud, virtuous and motivated society (Gibilisco, 2000:51). Amartya Sen portrays the mixed emotions of self-interest:

> 'Can you direct me to the Railway Station?' asks the stranger. 'Certainly,' says the local, pointing in the opposite direction to the post office, 'and would you post

this letter for me on your way?' 'Certainly,' says the stranger, resolving to open it to see if it contains anything worth stealing (Sen, cited in Stretton and Orchard, 1994:51).

During an interview with me, Hugh Stretton explained his dissent from this ideological interpretation of Adam Smith. He pointed out that Smith never said that the interests which prompted people's economic decisions and behaviour were all selfish. Smith's first book *The Theory of Moral Sentiments* was about our feelings, and concerns about other people's needs, safety and happiness, as well as our own. When he said in *The Wealth of Nations* that he owed his breakfast to his baker's self-interest, there is good reason to think that Smith meant the baker's joy in his skills and work, and pride in the quality of his bread and the pleasure it could give its consumers, as well as the money it earned him.

Smith certainly believed that people's generous feelings, and concern for others' safety and prosperity as well as their own, could join in determining their market choices and their social and political values and behaviour. Because it comes from the neoliberal 'bible' (i.e. Smith's *The Wealth of Na-*

tions) I think this observation must play a vital part of any effective attack on the neoliberals' assumption that material self-interest is the sufficient cause of market efficiency, which in turn, they then suggest, is a necessary condition (and many think a sufficient condition) of a good society.

The last 25 years have seen a revival in classical liberal ideals. Some people believe that Friedman and John Maynard Keynes are the most influential economists of the 20th century, although Friedman's free market seems to be winning traction over Keynes and his advocacy of government intervention.

It is, however, monetarism that is represented in the published and empirical works of 1974 Nobel Laureate in Economic Science, Milton Friedman. Friedman's professionalism has been highlighted by his marketised policy approach. He is best known for pointing out that stability in the growth of the money supply is crucial to controlling inflation and recessions, which not only raises questions about the government's control of money supply, but also of any one national government's ability to control trade in international finance and prevent increasing poverty, particularly in economies that have to purchase so-called hard currencies.

Friedman and other theorists of neoliberalism argue that their economic systems are to be produced by 'monetarist' means. Monetarism attributes interest rates, inflation, the level of output and prices to the velocity of money supply. Therefore, by giving stimulus to the nation's levels of aggregate demand the nation will act to increase the supply of money and, therefore, reduce interest rates. Monetarism is able to supply a route by which monetary policy can directly affect output and prices. In other words, monetarism is the study of the velocity of money supply.

However, there is an argument that Friedman's monetarism was created as a vehicle for the further development of the classical liberal doctrine, concerning the natural rate of unemployment. This is the idea that the economy tends to an equilibrium rate of unemployment at which the rate of inflation is stable. Friedman and most of his followers argue that any attempt to reduce the rate of unemployment beyond this level, through policies such as Keynesian demand management, will only further increase the rate of inflation without there being any real long-term increases in output or in rates of employment. Neoliberalism thereby rejects the goal of creating full employment through demand management.

Stretton has noted the political emergence of neoliberalism in Australia during the 1970s in these terms:

> Other interests saw opportunities to change the direction of development: to improve the mixed economies' efficiency by means which would incidentally make the rich richer, business freer, welfare cheaper and the poor more self-reliant. Those means were described as deregulating, privatising, restoring competition, cutting welfare, rolling back the boundaries of government (Stretton, 1987:7–8).

A critique of the economic ideology and theory behind neoliberalism

Marta Russell highlights the persistent inequalities that exist in the ideology and theory of classical liberalism and today's form of neoliberal economics. Neoliberalism and classical liberalism identify themselves with the position that, as the economy expands, everybody will share in its prosperity. Neoliberal economists believe social progress is merely a by-product of economic growth (Russell, 1998a; Orchard, 1989). They also argue, further, that neoliberal economics is capable of affecting nearly every facet of social life. For example, in the past 25 years neoliberal reforms have affected not only the economic lives of individuals, but have had a direct impact on the social lives of many people. Since its inception around the world, neoliberalism has widened the income gap between rich and poor, and created insecurities within the nature of work. Neoliberal politics has also brought about a poor quality and inflexible source of public services by reducing, restructuring and reforming government and its link to public services.

So why are neoliberal policies pursued? Advocates of neoliberalism say it aims to achieve progress by combining the operation of a free market with measures of social justice, in particular focused around the concept of meritocracy, which will, at least in theory, also contribute to economic growth. This view claims that the political motivation behind the neoliberal political actions enforces a new form of meritocracy. That is, to increase the effectiveness and efficiency of a market-driven economy neoliberals have introduced what is, theoretically, to be a global form of meritocracy.

More critical views have been widely expressed, arguing that this claimed form of equity is flawed, creating deep inequalities of outcome that threaten social cohesion, and that the neoliberal version of meritocracy only offers shifting patterns of inequality, unfairly exalting the rich, while condemning the poor to false hopes of individualised social mobility.

So it is worth further probing what 'meritocracy' means in theory and practice. Meritocracy is defined by government policies promoting the principles of merit. The actions pursued by advocates of meritocracy are fundamental to the belief that people get out of the system what they put into it, based on what they deserve, according to market-based principles. This is a political vision for the future based on merit, opposed to the traditionally conservative theories of the aristocracy. However, there are those who argue that this is just as bad because it allows people to acquire merit while not recognising that there are those who are born with the ability to acquire it and those who aren't, for example people with disabilities. This is, of course, detrimental to those with disabilities because the rich and powerful may arrogantly believe they fully deserved what they had, and that it was for the common good, however ruthless they were in achieving this 'merit'.

As a result, today, we may have the worst of both worlds. The rich are getting richer, while the poor are getting poorer. In the case of people with disabilities, their capacities under such a system are rarely deemed worthy of reward as being meritorious.

Neoliberalism in practice

In practice, neoliberal policies tend to encourage monopolies, rather than free market competition. At the same time they seek to maintain necessary global aspects of supply side economic reform to ensure an emphasis is placed on the government attaining a budget surplus and economic growth (Carlton, 2002).

The provision of public and collective social goods is provided by the government through the assistance of collective taxation. Economic liberalism affected not only the explicit institutions of the welfare state like social welfare benefits, but also the implicit contracts between workers and employers, under which employers would seek to preserve jobs— except in circumstances where the viability of their business was threatened—and to reward the loyalty of long-term employees through the maintenance of career paths. As John Quiggin puts it:

> From the 1980s onwards, businesses routinely dismissed employees in large numbers, not as a last resort, but as a preferred method of making already substantial profits even larger (Quiggin, 2009:6).

Industrial relations are one of the few areas of public policy where the Liberals and the Australian Labor Party can be seen to hold different agendas. Traditionally, the Liberals have represented the interests of business, particularly small business, while the Australian Labor Party is still largely dominated by trade unions. According to neoliberal philosophy, the issue of individualised workplaces has become highly politicised, delivering uncertainty for business as workplace agreements.

The United States and United Kingdom governments, led by Ronald Reagan and Margaret Thatcher respectively, during the 1980s delivered neoliberal reforms to public policy. In practice they delivered these reforms during a time when, they argued, there was a need for a new approach to government public policy. These governments approved the systematic pursuit of reduced public spending on welfare and allowed for tax cuts to the wealthy and corporations. They also raised money by selling publicly owned property and services. Such reforms to the public sector delivered an explicit economic message: survival of the fittest, there is no alternative. This became the driving force behind tough monetary targets. As Russell argues:

> They heralded the 'free' market as the salvation for all social ills (Russell, 1998b:168).

A key focus of neoliberal economics that focuses on both poor and rich nations is the privatisation of publicly owned assets and services by selling them to private investors, which is designed to phase out public programmes and to renounce government responsibility for social welfare.

Jim Carlton, former minister in the Liberal–National government (1975–1983), is an advocate for neoliberal economic reform, including the privatisation of state-owned assets. In an interview with me, Carlton argues that privatisation of state assets provides governments with an economic bonus, claiming that a shift from public to private allows the asset to capture all the competitive strategies that increase the profit margins, such as placing the emphasis on profit rather than on public need. Therefore, the government gains economically, because converting a service from public to private will also allow the government to collect company tax from it (Carlton, 2002). However, it can be argued that, while the neoliberal financial regime may have crumbled, the political agenda to defer authority to the market remains the same.

Is neoliberalism an answer to the challenges of globalisation?

After the Great Depression and World War II, some familiar big issues were on the agenda: protectionism, immigration, failing economies and economic nationalism. Our current headlines are dominated by similar concerns, so the question for political parties will be whether or not they can identify the wider trends and fashion effective policy responses in time to stave off conflict.

Globalisation processes have produced a world in which we live with the constant threat and reality of war that has created national tensions and conflicts. Peace was the promise of globalisation but terrorism and war is what we have inherited, while also providing us with increased poverty, economic insecurity and social exclusion.

The era of globalisation has introduced climate change, economic crises, crime and illegal drugs, terrorism, weapons of mass destruction, poverty, genocide, and human rights abuses. Complex global problems like these need global solutions. This suggests a need for the excluded to be more integrated into global society, or an alternative way to lead people out of poverty. Global economic redistribution could help to solve economic poverty.

The past global political agenda was structured by market-driven neoliberal reform. This is exemplified by the situation where the government will seek to reduce public expenditures to a level acceptable to financial markets. The equilibrium of financial markets is argued to be a global pursuit. Therefore, global pursuits are aligned, in many ways, to the political and economic market-driven actions of neoliberalism. This perspective argues that the easiest way to reduce government spending is by reducing social expenditure, but this simply results in placing extra burdens on the weak and the vulnerable.

Individualism has increasingly been able to drive home its economic benefits, becoming the favoured political perspective promoted by globalisation. However, globalisation also brings to the forefront a debate concerning uncertainty for the future of humanity. But the implications of the practice of globally inspired economic strategies are unjustifiable in the view of many pragmatic social democrats. These global market-driven strategies, as argued by Stretton and Stilwell, do not work to foster egalitarianism and social cohesiveness. By generating a cultural exposure to the politics of individualism, and linking it to the drive towards private economic wealth, the continual changes wrought by globalisation have simply confirmed and exacerbated structural inequality and social insecurity. It is no longer realistic to believe in the so-called 'trickle-down effect', since it just does not happen (Stretton, 1999). Money from the rich will rarely find its way into poorer hands, and certainly not in adequate amounts.

The global economic crisis can be attributed to the irrational assumptions underlying neoliberalism. This was in part attributed to the mistakes of post-war social democratic policy, so '[i]t is important that a resurgent social democracy should avoid repeating those mistakes' (Quiggin, 2009:13). A global political economy must have scope to improve facets of domestic financial regulation that are subject to irregular devices created through unregulated global financial markets. Global financial markets must be regulated and controlled. That is, there is a need for a reversal of global financial regulation to limit the possibility for compromises concerning domestic regulation, thereby fostering trade and investment and enhancing global financial markets, instead of undermining domestic regulation (Quiggin, 2009:13).

Neoliberalism and people with disabilities

Neoliberalism's agenda emphasises cost cutting and the privatisation of social security provision and public pension systems. Society imposes complex pressures upon nations to become part of the neoliberal political agenda. That is, while neoliberalism has respect for the design and structure of social insurance, including public pension systems, it is part of a conservative process to reduce and reform. Russell argues that neoliberal and third-way politics have much in common in this respect:

> That cuts to the quick of the neoliberal and Third-Way
> politics which have placed all the emphasis on ending

dependency and increasing productivity without any attention to equality of income which is directly tied into the freedom to live one type of life or another. Both replace redistributive (egalitarian) goals with a market approach; both adopt the supply-side theory that the economy is burdened by rigid labour markets, powerful trade unions, and [what they believe to be] overly-generous welfare provisions (Russell, 2001c:2).

Russell focuses on the social exclusion resulting from neo-liberal policy towards people with disabilities, with such exclusion resulting from the neoliberal conception that people with disabilities are non-compliant with a profit-making agenda. Most people with disabilities, according to a competitive neoliberal agenda, carry with them burdensome stigmas and disabilities that create problems for the social cohesion of society.

This lack of empathy shown in the Australian neoliberal agenda towards people with disabilities was highlighted by the Disability Reform Bill, introduced to Parliament in 2002 by the Liberal–National government led by John Howard. Its principal concern was with the blow out in costs of the disability services pension, and it was driven by the Howard government's 'reform' agenda for social spending. Such reforms sought to reduce social payments to people with disabilities and to strengthen their incentives to earn an income for a full week's work, instead of part-time work that entitles people with disabilities to a part pension including a pension card. The Bill would allow the Department of Family and Community Services to end both the allowance of a part pension and, more importantly, the desperately required pensioner benefits card, to those people with disabilities who are considered fit enough to work 15 hours or more per week. At that time, this Bill would have moved those people with disabilities onto an unemployment benefit that was reduced by $54-a-fortnight. Even though the Bill was defeated in the Senate in August 2002, the evident lack of empathy for the plight of people with disabilities can be seen as a hallmark of neoliberal policy.

During the previous electoral period from 2004–2007 the former Howard Liberal government had majority control of both houses of parliament, and was expected to reintroduce the 2002 Bill. The impact of such a Bill on people with disabilities was widely regarded as likely to be not only financially negative, but also socially, psychologically and culturally regressive.

The reason why the opposition parties blocked this Bill from passing through the Senate was because they, and ACOSS, didn't agree with the government's analysis that it was too easy to get a pension. In 1990 there were 300 000 people in receipt of the disability pension, and by 2002 the figure had risen to 650 000. Contrary to the government's argument that this increase revealed that the disability pension was too easy to access, ACOSS argued that a number of other reasons were involved.

The increase in numbers was partly created by the lack of access to other social security payments. For example, ACOSS released a report titled *Key causes for the rise in disability pensioners*. ACOSS claims that '[t]his research shows that in the late 1990s, [as an example] women's eligibility for the Age Pension was raised above 60 years and many mature-aged women with disabilities had to apply instead for a [disability pension]' (ACOSS, 2002a:1). ACOSS also argued that the government had not accounted for the rise in the number of people with disabilities entering the workforce. ACOSS suggested that 'likely reasons for this include the ageing of the population with mature age people being more likely to have disabilities; improved identification of disabilities such as mental illness; and improved care and treatment that has improved life expectancy rates for people with disabilities such as head injury.'

ACOSS also argued that the increase in numbers had been influenced by labour market factors, such as the recession, whereby 'during and after the recession of the early 1990s, many people became jobless and those with disabilities and related workforce barriers, such as age and limited skills, faced greater difficulty securing jobs' (ACOSS, 2002a:1). As ACOSS acknowledged, recessionary times have helped employers to focus on the stigmas and disutilities of the disabled body, reinforcing the stereotypical view that hiring people with disabilities hinders production and overall profits. This has been more recently acknowledged in a broad government publication that deals with issues confronting people with disabilities:

> It restricts the humanity of people with disability to reduce their much needed payment of support. This puts

the lives of the recipients of Disability support in to fear and desperation. Most disability support recipients are concerned about the possibility of the government reducing or ceasing social security/disability support (*Shut Out*, 2009:35).

This horrifying issue for many people with disabilities may again be on the neoliberal agenda. For example, in the 2010 election campaign the leader of the Coalition, Tony Abbott, pledged to reduce government spending by $47 billion. It is something that he believes will take pressure off interest rates. Does this mean there is a possibility that disability funding will also take a cut as it is part of government spending? Further to this Bill Shorten, Leader of the opposition announced on 25 October, 2013 that the National Disability Insurance Scheme may soon be privatised, voiding Coalition election promises.

Other aspects of the policy agenda in the last decade indicate further problems, particularly, the proposed welfare–pension reforms by the Coalition. Prior to the October 2004 federal election, a federal Coalition cabinet submission concerning welfare was leaked. The plan was that more than one million

Australians would have their, necessary, disability pension payments eroded. This was part of a secret Coalition bid to save money. The leaked submission of the federal Coalition argued that the current social security system undermines the policy goal of increasing labour market participation and that it is in the best interests of the Coalition parties to fix the welfare–pension problem immediately, as each year of delay will result in greater costs to the state. At the time, the government was spending about $24 billion a year on working-age income support, with the cost rising by about $1.5 billion each year. The leaked cabinet submission highlighted the problem that, since 1997, pension payments had been locked in at 25 per cent of average male weekly earnings, while allowances have always been linked to changes in inflation. Instead, the submission urged cabinet to 'seriously consider' the indexation arrangements, suggesting that the government's guarantee to maintain pensions at 25 per cent of male earnings should be abandoned. The submission stated that such welfare payments should be merged with Newstart and Youth Allowance to enable a single working-age welfare payout, saving the government about $1.3 billion.

To succeed in reducing the economic disadvantage and the

discrimination facing people with disabilities, the economic system must undergo serious practical changes, which will allow for an ethical and social focus on people with disabilities in society. Neoliberal economic processes are a contributing factor in the backlash against the social-policy agenda, blaming the poor structure and enforcement of such policies for the failure of people with disabilities to seek social inclusion and find work. The result of the dominance of neoliberal political economics has been continual rising inequalities.

Neoliberalism, marginalisation and social exclusion

It is pertinent to note the uproar that arose when the Business Council of Australia rather thoughtlessly spoke out about stripping the disability pension as an alternative to a flood levy to help the hardship suffered by the State of Queensland's flood victims. Disability advocates denounced this call.

The action proposed by the Business Council is yet another instance of policies based on the agenda of the neoliberal ideology. Political movements that advocate reforms, which allegedly simplify the process of benefit distribution, freely appeal to a need to reduce services, cut costs and for this the privatisation of public pension systems is all part of the plan.

There are already complex pressures on nations to become part of the neoliberal political agenda, and this proposal simply endorses those pressures by adding another example of 'cost cutting' here for redistribution there, all in the national interest.

That is, while neoliberalism is concerned with the design and structure of social insurance, including public pension systems, it is part of a conservative process to reform by particular kinds of reductions. Or, as Russell puts it:

> Neoliberal and Third-Way politics [...] have placed all the emphasis on ending dependency and increasing productivity without any attention to equality of income which is directly tied into the freedom to live one type of life or another. Both replace redistributive (egalitarian) goals with a market approach; both adopt the supply-side theory that the economy is burdened by rigid labour markets, powerful trade unions, and [what they believe to be] overly-generous welfare provisions (Russell, 2001).

Russell focuses on the social exclusion resulting from neo-liberal policy towards people with disabilities, and concludes that the exclusion that results is a direct outcome of the neo-liberal belief that people with disabilities are not compatible with a profit-making agenda.

Most people with disabilities, according to a competitive neoliberal agenda, carry with them burdensome stigmas and disutilities that create problems for the social cohesion of society. To some, the politics of the third-way, apparently, means that giving people with disabilities less will somehow empower them more. Obviously it is better to be in the work-force—better mentally, physically and psychologically—but if you don't have that option then how is it supposed to be OK to lose your financial safety net?

People with disabilities face this dilemma every waking moment of their day. It should be a priority for governments to provide social inclusion; new legislation must not close doors to the subsistent life that disability support pensions provide, but open doors for more people with disabilities to gain and keep jobs. Being a long-term unemployed person is not good for anyone's psychology and recovery. Yet, if the government is serious about finding more work for people with disabilities, they should not be looking to cut disability pensions. After all, people with disabilities are among the most impoverished unemployed and socially excluded peoples in society. This is acknowledged in the Australian government's (ALP) *Shut Out* report, as mentioned previously.

There is always a case for re-examining the construction of the disability pension, but the proposal to reduce the disability pension to pay for the flood levy, for example, is indicative of government's failure to adequately face the responsibility of providing needed assistance for people with disabilities. A compassionate society cares for its vulnerable members and provides an adequate standard of living.

At present, in Australia, there is an ongoing debate about the National Disability Insurance Scheme and how it should be funded. The present Liberal–National Government led by Tony Abbott is pushing to have the NDIS funded from general revenue; however, having it funded through a Medicare-style levy would ensure similar collectivist equality that over the years has pragmatically worked for funding health services.

Vern Hughes, an important political figure in the disability sector, believes the current NDIS proposal has features consistent with neoliberal ideology, which, he says, can be seen in the underlying assumptions of the scheme that gives its central attention to the impact upon the paid workforce and the overall health of the economy, rather than justifying the scheme in terms of its social role and the impacts it can be expected to make upon relationships of the people involved (Gibilisco, 2008).

The New Zealand approach

The experience of similar policies across the Tasman is also relevant. New Zealand's experience of universal disability insurance is centred on the role of the Accident Compensation Corporation (Gibilisco, 2008). The ACC has been in place for 38 years and is funded by small levies on motor vehicle registration, and on all workers. It covers all New Zealanders injured by accident whether they are earners or not. This system covers all medical expenses, rehabilitation, technology, disability support, wage compensation, and even the treatment needed for trauma from witnessing something horrific. In 2008, there was a push from neoliberal governments to privatise the scheme. We, therefore, need to ask: when we get a national disability insurance scheme in Australia, will it be a publicly or privately run agenda? Even with New Zealand's long-standing and well-managed State-initiated scheme, there is a push for privatisation of government-owned assets; it seems to be an enduring feature of public policy changes around the world.

In reality, though, there is no reason for the privatisation of the ACC. Such a move would simply transfer wealth from the government to private insurance companies. These plans are unnecessary and unfair as the ACC has not made a loss since the 1980s, is presently making surpluses, and has huge reserves.

Why can't we learn from the New Zealand experience and see the intense benefits of such a public insurance scheme? But if we here continue to ignore this possibility and push aside the calls for a publicly-funded and managed NDIS, then we will still be left with the substantial unmet need for disability services in the Australian disability sector. I personally have lived on my own for the past 21 years, with my severely progressive disability, without ever being privileged to receive the required amount of disability support as a matter of right.

My point is that we need an NDIS. But my question is this: what kind of NDIS will result? Will it meet personal and social needs, or will it just prove to be another neoliberal political tool—just a house built on sand?

Works Consulted

ACOSS (2002), 'Governments contribute to rise in Disability
Pensioners: new analysis', Media Release, 1–2,
http://www.acoss.org.au/dsp.htm.

Carlton, J. (2002), Interview with Peter Gibilisco, unpublished.

Gibilisco, P. (2008a), Feedback Forum: Universal access to
disability services defines our progress, *On Line Opinion*,
http://www.onlineopinion.com.au/view.asp?article=82
31&page=1.

Gibilisco, P. (2010), 'Neoliberalism and Impoverishment',
On Line Opinion, August 5, 1–2,
http://www.onlineopinion.com.au/view.asp?article=10
770.

Gibilisco, P. (2011f), 'Neoliberalism degrades disabled', *On
Line Opinion*, February 22, 1–2,
http://www.onlineopinion.com.au/view.asp?article=11
647.

Gibilisco, P. (2011h), 'The National Disability Insurance Scheme: friend or foe?', *On Line Opinion*, April 18, 1, http://www.onlineopinion.com.au/view.asp?article=11 915.

Hursh, D. (2003), 'Neoliberalism and schooling in the U.S, 'How state and federal government education policies perpetuate inequality', *Journal for Critical Education Policy*, Volume 1, Number 2, downloaded to Word, pp. 1–17, http://www.jceps.com/index.php?pageID=article&artic leID=12.

Orchard, L. (1989), 'Public Choice Theory and the Common Good', *Markets, Morals and Public Policy*, Orchard, L. and Dare, R. (eds), The Federation Press, Annandale, pp. 265–281.

Quiggin, J. (2009), 'An agenda for Social Democracy', *Perspectives*, Whitlam Institute, April 6, 1–16, http://www.whitlam.org/whitlam/images/whitlam_pers pectives_1.pdf.

Russell, M. (1998a), *Autobiography*, The MIT Press.

Russell, M. (1998c), 'Persistent Inequalities', *DisWeb: socio/economic aspects of disablement*, pp. 1–5, downloaded to Word, http://disweb.org/marta/pov.html.

Russell, M. (2001), 'Disablement, Oppression, and the Political Economy'. *Reinterpreting Disability Rights: Corporealities, Discourses of Disability*. University of Michigan Press, 1–35, http://www.martarussell.com/russell_umich_edit.html.

Shut Out (2009) 'Poverty and the Cost of Living with Disabilities', Commonwealth of Australia, 34–37.

Smith, A. (1976 [1776]), edited by Cannan E., An Inquiry into the Nature and Causes of: The Wealth of Nations, Cannan's Edition Originally Published in 1904 by Methuen & Co Ltd, University of Chicago Press, Chicago.

Stretton, H. (1987), *Political Essays*, Georgian House, Melbourne.

Stretton, H. (1999), *Economics a New Introduction*, UNSW Press, Sydney.

Stretton, H. (2003), Interview with Peter Gibilisco, unpublished.

Stretton, H. (2007), Interview with Peter Gibilisco, unpublished.

Stretton, H. and Orchard, L. (1994), *Public Goods, Public Enterprise, Public Choice: Theoretical Foundations of the Contemporary Attack on Government*, St Martins Press, New York.

Ullmann, O. (2001), 'So, What's New?', *The International Economy*, Volume 15, Issue 2, pp. 1-10, downloaded to Word, http://infotrac.galegroup.com/itw/infomark/375/437/39 339878w4/purl=rc1_EAIM_0_A73232538&dyn=8!xr n_37_0_A73232538?sw_aep=unimelb.

CHAPTER 3

The Third-Way (Social Democracy):
Just Neoliberalism with a Smiley Face?

> The intellectual climate has changed quite dramatically over the last few decades, and the tables are now turned. The virtues of the market mechanism are now standardly assumed to be so pervasive that qualifications seem unimportant. Any pointer to the defects of the market mechanism seems to be, in the present mood, strangely old-fashioned and contrary to contemporary culture (like playing an old 78rpm record with music from the 1920s) (Sen, 1999:111).

The third-way is a political model that, its supporters argue, encapsulates the best of both old left and new right politics. As such, it is regarded by leading social theorist and third-way advocate, Anthony Giddens, as the rebirth of the social democratic tradition. The political notions of liberty, justice and freedom highlight the third-way, the strategies of which, according to Giddens, are based upon the theories of mutualism and communitarianism, foundations of ethical socialism and classical liberalism. In contrast, others argue that it is a mirage, where no choice needs to be made between socialism and capitalism, and there exists agreement between right and left.

This chapter seeks to make sense of this so-called third-way, by examining its origins, nature and influence. It then proceeds to a critical assessment of its significance for the welfare state, before turning to look in particular at the National Disability Insurance Scheme and how the third-way relates to people with disabilities.

Insights into the political economy of the third-way

Central to the third-way is its support of the neoliberal belief concerning markets, in particular, the idea that unfettered markets will benefit all of society. This belief has a profound effect on social-policy processes.

During the financial crisis of the 1930s, unemployment was rampant and many banks were driven to a state of collapse, losing millions from the savings accounts of depositors. The crisis was overcome in time, and, as a result, governments introduced strict regulations designed to ensure that banks had adequate funds and would not engage in high-risk ventures for the sake of profits. The resultant political economic strategy was to ensure that government-owned savings banks were available for low-income savers.

Economic liberals extended the move towards freer trade in goods and services that began with the Bretton Woods conference in 1944, and the establishment of the Global Agreement on Trade and Tariffs. With some relatively minor exceptions (such as attempts to undermine environmental protections and trade union rights in the name of free trade) the growth in trade in goods and services has been overwhelmingly beneficial, unlike the disproportionate expansion in financial flows. Any new international settlement must encourage trade and ensure that global financial markets facilitate trade and investment, rather than destabilising them. These lessons will be of particular importance when the economy emerges from the current crisis (Quiggin, 2009:13).

Political scientist Lionel Orchard argues that neoliberalism pursues the systematic political thought that the attainment of social and public good is a by-product of an unhindered approach to markets (Orchard, 1989:271). However, there is no logical reason for the marketisation of services essential for human conditioning, such as education, health and welfare. Rather, there is a need for essential human services to be provided on the basis of social justice, rather than being left to the economic principles of the market. The challenge for the third-way becomes one of balancing the market and social justice.

There is a view that the theoretical foundations of the third-way can be linked to the political success of the Hawke and Keating Australian Labor Party (ALP) governments in the period 1983–1996. The Hawke and Keating government's rule was believed by many political analysts to be a successful period for a social democratic government, and indeed its successful policies were benchmarked by other social democrats around the world.

During this period the ALP adopted policy strategies that were viewed as unorthodox by many traditional social democratic policy advocates. Policy reforms included the shrinking of the size of the State by allowing legislative deregulation of market activities and the selling, or tendering out, of State-owned assets. This included moving towards the privatisation of money-making government assets such as the

Commonwealth Bank, Commonwealth Serum Laboratories and Telecom, the deregulation of the banking sector, and the floating of the Australian dollar.

At the same time, in the US and the UK, Bill Clinton's and Tony Blair's version of political economic renewal was the acceptance globalisation within electoral politics. However, the public seems to be increasingly cynical about electoral politics within the spectrum of global politics, seeing decisions being made more on a global level than on a national, or even local level.

Such debates suggest that globalisation poses key questions for proponents of both the third-way and pragmatic social democracy.

The core principles of a third-way style of politics can be described as radical, while having the ability to update and achieve a policy mix that is more suitable for the social needs of contemporary societies. It is a system that promotes the collective pursuit of progressive income taxation that will help fund the methods of redistribution to ensure a greater equality of income and wealth. The third-way seeks to promote full employment through the process of market-driven economic growth, combining it with social democratic cra-dle-to-the-grave welfare to deliver basic human rights. Thus, it is argued, the third-way maintains many of the core social democratic principles that can help in the delivery of a so-cially just market economy. However, the third-way is much more market friendly than earlier forms of social democracy. The inherited traditions of post-World War II social democ-racy, it is argued, fail to meet the complex economic and so-cial needs of globalisation.

Lionel Orchard defines the third-way as being a theory that is much less pretentious than the traditional form of social de-mocracy, as it is supposed to uphold the political strengths of both neoliberalism and social democracy. Orchard argues that the third-way, in theory, is supposed to develop the social and economic security of society by using the public sector to countervail processes of the private market, promoting meth-ods that allow private means to supply social democratic ends. Such an approach views the private sector as an enhan-cer of collective good (Orchard, 2002).

A restructure and reform of past social democratic policies that were suitable for the post World War II period up to the

1970s is needed, without losing Labor values and beliefs.

It is evident that some of the theoretical objectives of the third-way justify social democratic recognition. For example, the third-way argues for the need to reconfigure the operation of public goods and services. Third-way theory acknowledges the need to question how the public sector is owned, operated, funded and delivered, so that its services can generate an abundance of socially driven values in the communities they serve.

The third-way requires that the role of government be fundamentally reformed to facilitate partnerships and cooperation by bringing together institutions and individuals in all areas of public policy. Cooperation will lead in turn to compassion.

Amitai Etzioni argues that a modern form of liberal politics that incorporates elements of communal and socialist political principles is the best form of political system to create a more inclusive society. Etzioni's style of communitarian politics is closely aligned to principles outlined in the third-way. He argues that liberal ideology can enhance individual freedom and respect, while ensuring and maintaining equality of opportunity for all people. For Etzioni, a system based on open market exchanges will allow the maintenance of economic freedom of choice while also creating equality of access, according to merit, to areas such as education and training. This system is based on meritocracy, and the argument that people get out of society what they put in. The third-way, in theory, claims to focus on social policy, which can repair unfair social effects of free-market economic policy. Its advocates talk of a mix of civic socialism and communitarian liberalism. This debate is seen in the following terms:

> There must be a secret prize for whoever comes up with the most dismissive epitaph for the third-way. This seems the only possible explanation for the torrent of phrases depicting it as 'vague', 'fuzzy', 'waffle', 'a masterwork of ambiguity' or, as the *Economist* had it: 'Trying to pin down an exact meaning is like wrestling an inflatable man. If you get a grip on one limb, all the hot air rushes to another' (Etzioni, 2001b:1).

Etzioni insists that the third-way is more than just modern rhetoric. He argues that it is a focused strategy for an economic age of globalism, one that sees many benefits in the prospect of free global trade.

The third-way, in part, rests on a system of civic responsibility. Civic responsibility recognises that you cannot renew a community by issuing a set of top-down instructions. There is a need for a community approach that can see the benefit gained in looking after society's most valuable assets, namely one another. A community that works towards the collective goals of a society is acting as a beacon for communal social cohesiveness.

According to this analysis, social entrepreneurs can be effective in providing state savings and responsibility, driving down the need for a large public sector. Social entrepreneurs are defined by some third-way thinkers as entrepreneurs who do not work towards individual profit, but who work, instead, towards the community benefit. Social capital is a key element in the success of the third-way, having no direct links with individual profit, and, therefore, is driven by the pursuits of social entrepreneurs. In the past, community development has either followed the production strategies of top-down or bottom-up processes. However, with the guidance

and assistance of social entrepreneurs, community development is likely to grow inside-out. This is the best way to foster and generate social capital, which in theory has a social
and economic equalising effect through society. The creation
of this social platform will allow government to achieve its
best results in the development of programs indirectly and
directly related to finance, employment and training.

Social entrepreneurialism has brought about change in the
current pursuits of global corporatism and political leaders. It
is said to have brought social development within the corporate sector into vogue. Think Richard Branson, or Bill Gates.
Social entrepreneurs exist in the space between the public
sector and the market, where both have failed to deliver important goods and services to those who can afford to pay
only a minimal amount. Social entrepreneurs may, or may
not operate for profit, but their main aim is that of social
transformation. This is often done by finding ways that develop the social inclusiveness of the corporate sector, while
adding to its profits. Taking this view forward, it can be argued that the purpose of government must be to bring institutions and individuals closer together, to create the circumstances by which cooperation between them becomes possi-

ble. There is a need to practise compassion of a collective kind. In this process, social entrepreneurs play a crucial part in modernising the nation, allowing nations to be competitive in a global structure.

Another fundamental aspect of the third-way is the responsibility of a third-way government to accept and continue the economic reform of the late 1970s to the present. This means reducing the size and power of the state to intervene in the unfettered freedom of markets, ensuring that markets are structured to pursue competition. Capital markets are mostly open to change, while labour markets can be seen as more flexible, and quick to adapt to an ever-changing workforce. The management of third-way policies requires a reduction in state intervention.

Lindsay Tanner, former Minister for Finance in the Federal Australian Labor Party government, is also a key third-way thinker. He argues that government regulation, as opposed to state ownership, must take a pivotal role, because private enterprise is more able to structure itself as an economic powerhouse. Therefore, the third-way, according to Tanner, views government regulation as a means to enforce social contracts on private companies (Tanner, 2002).

It is not the agenda of the third-way to argue that competition is best served by deregulation. The third-way views regulation as seeking to improve the operation of the market, not to replace, or impede it. It is a search for the correct balance between regulation and deregulation.

Some proponents of the third-way argue that third-way policies will lead to a more effective style of government, one that challenges the boundaries between government and business and allows government to be aligned with the contemporary world.

The third-way critique of the welfare state

Because of work done by people such as Anthony Giddens, the current ideology and intellectual structure of the third-way is now at the fore of social democratic politics. As an academic sociologist and a Fellow of Kings College Cambridge, he became the Director of the London School of Economics and Political Science. In fact he promoted himself as Tony Blair's (former UK prime minister) inspiring and favourite intellectual (see for example the front cover of Giddens, 2000). Indeed, Giddens' theories are recognised by politicians and intellectuals alike as key contributions to the development of the third-way as a political philosophy.

Giddens argues that we should move beyond traditional forms of social democracy in an attempt to modernise the theory. Giddens' approach is that social democratic political structures have to be reformed to bring about economic and social progress. By contrast, Nursey-Bray argues that the consequences of such reforms are a watered down form of social democracy that cannot maintain a humane form of social inclusion. He argues this is due to the third-way's heavy reliance on markets that put profit before people (Nursey-Bray, 2001).

A further argument is that the third-way's most fundamental action towards the attainment of equality is the promotion of equality of access. Equality of access is applied in circumstances that can assist those in pursuit of equality, which in theory becomes a means of enhancing social inclusion through equal forms of social mobility. Equality of access is both relevant and robust, avoiding both the theoretical drawbacks of equality of outcome and equality of opportunity.

Equality of access brings rationality to policies that involve equality, and is able to provide a benchmarked position by which to measure policies of equality.

This is a claim that equality of access provides a much needed fresh outlook on the problem of social exclusion. Equality of access isn't just about money, but is about all things that make for an enjoyable life and citizenship. Therefore, equality of access has the capacity to provide people with disabilities with a much more inclusive future. This approach identifies equality of access with the equalising of opportunities for individuals to generate income to attain an adequate standard of living. The global political development of reforms to welfare, imposed by the third-way and neoliberal government's welfare policies, are structured towards participation. That is, in third-way approaches most people of working age share in an obligation to participate in the workings of business, government and community. This reopens the debate about one's ability to participate and perform under structured or unstructured working conditions.

Mutual obligation implies that those who can work should do so, and should not seek welfare payments. The community must also hold up its end of the deal concerning mutual obligation, ensuring that the means to earn a decent living are available, and that employees are properly treated. The government also has a duty to supply pensions to the elderly and to people with disabilities, and the pensions should ensure an adequate standard of living. This is explicitly acknowledged in the third-way critique of neoliberalism.

In the last 30 years the welfare state has played a major role in creating a profound divide between left and right politics. Social democrats should accept some of the criticisms made by the right concerning the welfare state. The right argues that the welfare state is undemocratic because it depends on a top-down distribution of benefits. The welfare state is concerned about is protection and care, but in the process, fails to give enough recognition to personal liberty. The right also argues that welfare institutions are bureaucratic, alienating and inefficient. Not in total disregard of the right's criticisms of the welfare state, the third-way does not wish to dismantle the welfare state, but to reform it.

How Australia became reliant on the third-way

Australian politics has always maintained a very pragmatic

stance, and therefore did not pursue any of the benefits offered by traditional Marxist and European social democratic welfare policies. A shift towards a third-way form of politics in Australia was built upon electoral dissatisfaction with militant unions in the late 19th or early 20th centuries, although some say that Australian politics during that time lacked direction, failing to focus on the development of Marxist politics.

Such politics helped Australia in the creation of such legislation as the centralised wage fixing system, where wages move in combination with a liberalised market economy. During Deakin's time, in the 1890s and 1900s, Australia had the 'new protectionism' with its attendant inefficiencies. There have been many times in history that the ALP has been interested in reforming these traditional political systems, to enhance issues dealing with equality of opportunity, and to some degree to engage with the effectiveness and efficiency of society; however, such moves have also been suppressed by the mood of the Australian electorate and factional fighting in the ALP. The shackles of political history were finally abandoned by the ALP in the years of the Hawke and Keating governments when the ALP government's hand was forced by the global financial markets, and it took the courage to make the necessary reforms. The Hawke and Keating governments could be seen as an inspiration to left-wing parties internationally who wanted to gain or keep government. That is, left-wing parties around the world in the post-stagflation era saw merit in the ALP's approach to politics. And the ALP government was able to gain electoral support for five consecutive elections during the period from 1983 to 1996.

Thirty years have passed since the golden age of capitalism. However, in the intervening period, social democracy was still defined as Keynesianism plus the welfare state. Many third-way thinkers argue that we can still create a political program that is more relevant, robust and dynamic. The third-way has promoted a social, economic and political agenda that is able to meet the needs of a society vastly reliant on technological improvements, global trade, and the economic freedom of competition.

It can be argued that the welfare state has not operated to promote the social democratic ideals of collectivism. People who have a high level of social capital and self-esteem are more likely to use government training programs and social welfare. So, the success of the welfare state relies heavily on the success of civil society.

This should lead to a social democratic model where the state can provide the basis for social and communal cohesiveness, rather than the state being depicted as a paternalistic money tree. The provision of a third-way welfare state will not require the withdrawal of resources for the provision of welfare, but rather the aim will be to focus on redevelopment of welfare programs. Government policies should concentrate on giving power to classify, dispense and administer social action to those who show interest within the community, rather than to bureaucracies. However, many factors impede welfare. These include the market economies of the right and the bureaucratic administration of the left. Both have weakened society's claim to effective forms of collective action. Most forms of right-wing politics sanctify anything that will help to promote self-interest, which those on the right believe will drive home the supremacy of individual freedom and action. However, the left see such supremacy as a problem, and state-administered collectivism remains primarily a political economic objective of left-wing politics.

For all its achievements, however, the welfare state has not been good at creating collectivism. It has not fostered a feeling of mutual interest and support between people. It has, in fact, delivered an individualised form of compassion.

Social democratic politics has traditionally regarded the state as the arbiter of collective institutions. However, in practice, this has been a delusion, because most work is directed at individuals with payments made directly to them, rather than directing resources at communities.

The National Disability Insurance Scheme

A National Disability Insurance Scheme for people who experience catastrophic injury was an idea endorsed by the Australian 2020 summit (held in 2008) as a way to provide further funding for the disability services needed by this group of citizens in our community. This endorsement was made in the context of an overarching concern about funding for disability services at a national level. The NDIS proposes a strategy that would secure and develop new streams of funding for disability services. At present, the only forms of no-fault coverage for catastrophic injury are through the various WorkCover arrangements maintained by the states for those injuries acquired at work; and through no-fault transport accident schemes maintained by Victoria, New South Wales, Tasmania and the Northern Territory.

Outside these schemes, Australians suffering such injuries, for example, through transport accidents, domestic accidents, sporting injuries or assaults, are left high and dry. So, too, are those who acquire injuries due to a degenerative disease or a chronic illness, or who are born with a disability: they have no recourse to lifetime care and support outside the minimal assistance provided by the already overburdened and crisis-driven public disability assistance systems.

These facts alone make it clear why a strong correlation exists between disability and poverty—the costs associated with disability are substantial and, either directly or indirectly, delivers costs that, in terms of flow-on effects, every member of the community has to bear.

At present, the burden of caring for those with disabilities falls to families with assistance from State and Commonwealth governments. The cost of disability is already placing far too great a demand upon today's welfare system, and there is every probability that costs will continue to increase

significantly. One of the major factors driving this is the substantial increase in the number of people with disabilities. It
is believed that the Australian population will grow by three
million in the next 15 years and one estimate suggests that
two in every five of the future population increase will involve people with some kind of disability.

There are aspects of our current economic vision that are
global, and global forces are also driving the current crisis in
welfare provision. However, as proposed at the 2020 summit,
this could be alleviated by government action to reform the
way we deal with disability, as with the NDIS proposal. This
would be one way in assisting those engaged in the empowerment of the many Australians affected by disablement, and
it would be good for our society as a whole.

Such a scheme would allow all Australians to fulfil their aspirations for a way of life in which fair and just treatment is
available to all. Such a scheme would clarify Australia's
claim to be a 'fair-go' culture. Is there not a positive chance
that Prime Minister Tony Abbott's government can build on
the previous Gillard Labor government's proposal and bring
about such an effective social reform with insignificant costs

to the public at large?

Such a scheme would also give added substance to the Liberal Party's current commitment to the social inclusion of all Australians. Relying on family network of the person with a disability to provide the principal carer is not a long-term solution. The system's reliance upon family members is flawed. We must face the fact that family members are human; they get old, become sick and die. And the socioeconomic agenda of today's globally competitive environment has turned the ability of parents to be the primary carers of their disabled children upside down. Both parents need to work to pay the bills and this demand is not about to change in the situation caused by the recent financial turmoil.

There is likely to be an amplification of demand for support services within the disability sector, combined with the evident limits of family carers to provide care for their children and siblings with disabilities. And this will lead to the magnification of costs within disability support services, and only put further strains on the bottom line of government budgets.

In the 1980s there was a similar problem concerning the dependency of Australia's ageing population on the age pension, and the discovery that any continuation of the status quo in service provision would place intolerable demands on the taxpayer. Hence, the development of superannuation became a necessary and effective solution to this problem.

The NDIS should cost a meagre amount when shared across the entire population. That is, it should be funded through a Medicare levy, drawing on the processes of public equality outlined by the previous Labor Government. I for one hope the current Liberal–National coalition government can see the overwhelming need for such a scheme. This includes the pursuit of social justice and equality, which is made much easier by maintaining public ownership of the scheme. Therefore, in all likelihood, it would lead to more people in the paid workforce. It would also encourage an increase in general skill levels. Carers must be recognised and respected as providing an indispensable contribution.

This then would benefit economic growth in two ways: first, by vastly increasing disposable income within the community; and, second, it would reduce the benefits overall that governments have to pay. That is, such a move will provide for an increase in taxes paid, an increase in national productivity, and will help to reduce a looming workforce crisis.

The third-way and people with disabilities

A political analysis of the third-way is beneficial to people with disabilities.

Most third-way and neoliberal sympathisers conclude that meritocracy will tend to increase social mobility in a new era of equal opportunity, one that offers people every chance to fulfil their own potential (Gibilisco, 2009a). Dan Finn takes account of various difficulties faced by the third-way, in its handling of people with disabilities. Finn also acknowledges, however, that the third-way's approach to people with disabilities has made significant steps forward. Finn argues that third-way has been able to provide work for those who have the skills, while devising ways to increase the provision of such skills to people with disabilities. But Finn also argues that the application of such policies is fraught with difficulties—in the extension of meaningful employment rights and adequate benefits for workers with disabilities (Finn, 2002).

Such policy shifts will also require suitable fiscal funds to correct public policy and tackle the drift towards economic inactivity of people with disabilities (Finn, 2002). For example, people will say it is not their responsibility to be concerned about a disabled person's carer, or how they will get to work or class; it is all too hard.

Many people with disabilities suffer greatly from a severe lack of resources, thereby leading to a denial of equality of access to human rights and responsibilities. Such rights and responsibilities are those that will attempt to secure social cohesion and democratic participation leading to personal development. Adequate development of these policies will act to further ingrain the rights of people with disabilities that allow and promote most forms of social and economic participation and responsibilities in society. They further argue for an adequate form of income for people with disabilities that will allow for a decent standard of living.

There is potential to harness the mutual interests of people with disabilities. These mutual interests are able to develop a position from where we can build equal rights and equal access into the design of new services, products and buildings. Models of success for people with disabilities are dependent on the promotion of both new partnerships and disability rights. Such new partnerships are based on the mutual interest of disabled and non-disabled people, working together to bring disability rights to the centre of the political agenda. There are mutual benefits to be gained from an increase in social inclusion for people with disabilities by developing work, learning, citizenship and the design of the built environment to cater for all.

At the moment, products, services and the built environment all contribute to enforcing social exclusion upon people with disabilities, and acting as major barriers to their becoming fully functioning members of society. Such exclusion is related to discrimination and a lack of awareness of the challenges confronting people with disabilities. Factors such as technological advancement and new partnerships will assist through the next 10 to 15 years to promote unprecedented opportunities for people with disabilities and their organisations.

In other words, if you want it you must create it. This concept encapsulates the neoliberal and meritocratic political agenda. A political analysis of the third-way is beneficial to people with disabilities. In the approach of a meritocratic future, some argue that in the new political arena there will be no socialist or benevolent capitalist solutions to social policy; no one will do it for us, we will have to do it by ourselves.

In effect, government is seen as the last resort. But this discounts the collective ability of government and the public sector's abilities to provide a paradigm that can ameliorate the social and economic exclusion of people with disabilities. The individual person as the arbiter of their own past and destiny. This approach fails to place much hope in the potentially positive role of the state in promoting the rights of people with disabilities. This agenda suggests that there is an extended invisible hand in the marketplace to assist people with disabilities who want to make the move to a more inclusive future. But, as I establish throughout this book, market failure is one of the major contributors to the economic and social exclusion of people with disabilities. For example, in a competitive market system most businesses or companies cannot afford to delve into their profit margins in order to make the workplace more flexible and suitable for some people with disabilities.

To overcome the costs of neglect, some have suggested that it is important to invest in people with disabilities. But this statement is empty and meaningless if it is taken in isolation from the social complexity facing people with disabilities. It is only through the pragmatic and interrelated education of the nondisabled and people with disabilities alike that the neglect can be appreciated and transformed. The neglect shown by post-World War II social democracy had a profoundly negative effect on people with disabilities, such as the creation of institutions and negative stereotypes by social norms which arise from historically uneducated affiliations (Johnson, 2002). On the other hand, social democracy was developing the beginnings of the welfare state that has assisted in providing a space in which the politics of people with disabilities could move from the margins to the mainstream.

A system of meritocracy is one that is proactive about the politics of the third-way and people with disabilities, and which is currently in vogue thanks to third-way and neoliberal ideologies. As Russell puts it:

> Once the neoliberals and Third-Way politicos have been convinced they have done all they can do to help the disadvantaged seize their 'opportunities' and be-

come 'independent and productive' as [George Bush] puts it, the mood is likely to shift to blaming those disabled persons left on entitlement programs for their individual failure to make the grade—all the more reason to shave benefits to induce more incentives to the recalcitrant to get a job (Russell, 2001c:4).

Russell drives home a plausible political objective of both neoliberal and third-way governments, namely that they seek to reform, by which they mean reduce, the cost of the welfare state with regards to people with disabilities, and thus increase the chance for a government budget surplus.

President Barack Obama accepted the 2009 Nobel Peace Prize for his progressive approach to social policies. This commitment is also shown in his vision for including people with disabilities in social life. He set this out in one of his campaign speeches:

We must build a world free of unnecessary barriers, stereotypes, and discrimination ... policies must be developed, attitudes must be shaped, and buildings and organizations must be designed to ensure that everyone has a chance to get the education they need and live independently as full citizens in their communities (Obama, April 11, 2008 cited in White House—President, 2009:1).

In this speech, Obama highlighted some of his deep-down assumptions about a just society: it also must involve the inclusion of people with disabilities. Are Obama's progressive political theories demonstrating concern for people with disabilities? Have his resultant policies given expression to his vision of equality and the end of discrimination? He has shown his intention to create pathways to realise objectives, by ensuring an increase in funding for the enforcement of the *Americans with Disabilities Act* (White House—President, 2009).

High on Obama's agenda is the lifting of the employment rate among people with disabilities. To achieve this he plans to, first, require compliance in the American public sector to a wave of 'affirmative action' type legislation, to which people with disabilities will be the beneficiaries. The next phase of this agenda will be to implement such reforms in the private sector. Obama argues that policy should encourage those employers to use existing tax benefits to hire more workers with disabilities and support small businesses owned by people with disabilities (Gibilisco, 2009d).This connects with a political insistence on the rise of a new form of meritocracy, which can be prejudicial and, ultimately, discriminatory against those with socially defined lesser or different abilities. In particular, neoliberalism and the third-way carry with them a new form of meritocracy, in that the individualising tendencies of the merit principle, which have long existed in western democracies, are given further emphasis, for example, through policies such as 'mutual obligation'. In the context of neoliberalism and the third-way, merit can now be used as a means of blaming individuals for their supposed failures and of removing the focus from the broader societal context in which people live. In essence, under the current individual-focused approach of neoliberal and third-way policy, meritocracy results in the exacerbation of merit as a concept that carries a biomedical assumption of worth and value as being able bodied; this supposition is narrowly defined, thereby excluding all those labelled as living with a disability. Meritocracy is the major difference between old world classical liberalism and the global stylings of neoliberalism.

Global forms of politics, according to neoliberal political

sources, are said to have moved beyond traditional methods of equal opportunity, thereby increasing the social mobility and inclusion of people with disabilities. What one is born with, or without, is not of one's own doing; or to put it in a more crude form of discourse, being a member of the 'lucky sperm club' confers no moral right to advantage.

To give further backing to the pledge that the global era will create more societal inclusion for people with disabilities, we can point to Gordon Brown who was Blair's successor as prime minister and leader of the Labour Party in the UK. In 2006, Gordon Brown was named the UK's most influential disabled person by *Disability Now* newspaper. He suffers from a vision impairment caused by a rugby injury in his teenage years, and, hence, he qualified for nomination and was chosen from a list of 25 finalists that included physicist Dr. Stephen Hawking.

However, the question remains, does the fact that Gordon Brown has vision impairment, and is the father of a child with cystic fibrosis, influence his and his party's policies and, therefore, world politics?

In Australia, the previous 2007–2013 Federal ALP government, previously led by former prime minister Kevin Rudd, undertook important initiatives. These have been followed by Bill Shorten, the former parliamentary secretary for disabilities and children services, who is seeking to reduce the stigmas created by neoliberal global social and economic reform. In a speech to the Western Australian Disability Collective, Shorten spoke optimistically about the political processes concerning disability:

> In politics, there is no premium on bad news. The premium is on the good news, the announcables, the releases, the positive stories, but I believe in disability if we're to move to the positive, taking nothing away from the many accomplishments of many people over many years and decades, we have to promote and recognise the bad news (Shorten, 2009:10).

The present leader of the ALP Bill Shorten in a previous speech was quick to point out, as an Australian politician, that Australians are not malicious. Unfortunately though, we still have a two-class society when it comes to disability and impairment. As Shorten adds: 'Like all prejudice, prejudice against people with impairments is an opinion not sustained by any fact. In fact, it is born of ignorance and a lack of empathy for the experiences of others' (Shorten, 2009:13).

As a government that claimed to be progressive in a global sense, the immediate aim of the approach adopted by Rudd's administration was to inform, interview, collaborate and compromise with most stakeholders in the disability sector. For example, with the lowest rates of employment among people with a disability on the OECD, the former Rudd government wished to more fully understand why people with disabilities found it so hard to participate in the workforce; after all participation in work is empowering.

Writing about Australian policies towards people with disabilities, Mike Clear and Brendan Gleeson contend that an increase in the social and economic exclusion of people with disabilities has been created by flawed neoliberal welfare reforms (Clear and Gleeson, 2002:37). Such reforms are structured to attain a systematic reduction in cost to the government, at least in ratio per population. Such reforms usually do not take into account that people with disabilities are human, too, suffering from an infinite number of actions and behaviours that cannot be stereotyped for cost-benefit reasons (Gibilisco, 2004a; 2004b; Russell, 2001b; 2001c; Stretton, 2003).

The third-way in practice

The third-way is not a political ideology separate from economic and social policies of government. It is about rights and responsibilities, but it is also about public administration and management, in particular economic management. As former British prime minister Tony Blair claimed, you cannot be a government that redistributes wealth and opportunity unless you're running a strong, fiscally disciplined economy.

More critical analysts, by contrast, argue that third-way governments have continued, and gone beyond, the neoliberal policies of their conservative predecessors, such as Reagan and Thatcher. For example, in practice, the third-way's focus upon monetary policy as the driving force behind market-driven capitalism has helped the continued growth of social and economic inequality (Russell, 2000a; Stretton, 1996).

It is disappointing, but not surprising to many of the UK's traditional Labour voters, that the level of inequality in the UK has increased under New Labour. However, Blair believes that the UK needs a more meritocratic society, one based on the notion of equality of access. He is of the opinion that a more meritocratic state is the essence of his policies towards equality of access that will be beneficial to UK society by providing a system of equal worth. Meritocracy in many circumstances is a product of the merit attained from education and training. Education and training is argued to be the key to many forms of social mobility in today's society. Meritocracy is structured according to education and training opportunities, and assisted by a program of equality of access to such programs.

Linked to this, Blair argued that the third-way is about reasserting New Labour as a party of values, and rediscovering a belief in community, opportunity and responsibility. But now what remains of the third-way? What is the political legacy left by the Blair Labour government in the UK? Many believe that the Labour Party's crowning achievement was the death of politics. Yes, some believe, Britain is in a better place than when they took over government, but the veneer has worn off and there is nothing left to vote for.

Tony Blair's initial election victory was in 1997. Following this, Blair's parliamentary rule was filled with the general public's high hopes, expectations of goodwill and good, progressive political leadership. However, a consideration of opinion polls after 10 years painted a very different picture. By 2007, opinion polls showed that only 11 per cent of voters liked him, with 57 per cent believing he stayed on too long.

Blair's leadership was one that was characterised by political turmoil; he was said to be an inspiring leader of his team, but by the end of his term his cloak of authority was totally threadbare. During Blair's time in office, community attitudes changed, giving rise to selfishness and morally inhumane acts, spearheading other changes across society. He will be remembered primarily for his alliance with the United States on Iraq, and for the unfulfilled promises made in 1997.

The upbeat selling of third-way social democracy went off the boil with the departure of Tony Blair. The 2007 victory of the ALP in Australia did little to restore it, since the third-way approach had been so closely linked to the beliefs of the former ALP leader Mark Latham. When Kevin Rudd, former prime minister, gained power, he sought to denounce neoliberalism, but largely avoided embracing the third-way rhetoric. But critical discussion of the underlying assumptions of the third-way social-policy agenda is still highly relevant; and this chapter argues that such historical discussion will help in our assessment of Rudd's policies in Australia, Gordon Brown's agenda after Blair in the UK, and even Barack Obama's welfare policy strategies in the US. This essay is an historical contribution to that necessarily critical discussion of the assumptions underlying social policy. Has the situation that the third-way terminology tried to address changed all that much just because it has gone off the boil? Of course not. The rhetoric may no longer attract attention but to suggest that examination of its assumptions is outdated ignores the social-policy facts: those assumptions are still alive and need to be critically discussed (Wearne, 2009).

However, as revealed in this chapter, the theoretical principles of social democracy contained within the third-way are ultimately diminished to the point of not being implemented. In particular, the empowering potential of the third-way is continually challenged and undermined by its reliance on market mechanisms to promote social policy. The outcome for people with disabilities is a situation whereby their social exclusion is exacerbated through policies ultimately focused on cost cutting and seeking to produce budget surpluses, resulting in severe limitations on what the social policies provide.

Can the third-way's form of social democracy on its own harmonise globalisation?

A social democratic response to the crisis must begin by reasserting the crucial role of the state in risk management. If individuals are to have security of employment, income and wealth, governments must establish the necessary legal and economic framework and enforce its rules (Quiggin, 2009:5).

The global financial crisis has created and developed the conditions in which a new social democratic agenda can be realistically put forward. That is, the new system of social democracy will be changed to incorporate global complexities, while maintaining the political, social and economic logical standpoint that has emerged as a result of the global financial meltdown (Quiggin, 2009:4).

Unlike the failed third-way version of social democracy this new form will not have to align itself with a neoliberal political economy. Thus, the social democratic tradition can draw upon valid and socially beneficial reasons for reform, as we face the new challenges and constraints arising after the collapse of the economic order that, for three decades, was said to replace everything that had preceded it (Gibilisco, 2009c:3).

In the past, when facing a financial crisis, traditional social democratic policy would have focused upon financial and macroeconomic management that in turn dealt with the national and international banking system. Such a policy can provide the most effective stimulus to the economy at both international and national levels. That is, the delivery of social and economic good that comes out of the global financial crisis may promote radical transformations in political decisions to bring about the most pragmatic transformation of social life (Quiggin, 2009:5–6; Gibilisco; 2009c:3).

Adding to this, there are two points of view: One position is held by those who believe the financial market needs better transparency, and that stability should be the focus, whereas equality is secondary. It is a position that can be typified by the theory and analyses of the third-way. Such a political device was developed to deal with the complexities of globalisation and justified its approach by aligning itself to the neoliberal ideal of increased individual freedom, maximising choices, and enhanced equality of opportunity. It thus favoured light regulation, limited by its focus on macroeconomic stability, while leaving markets to play the larger role in the global economy. The other position, where lightly or unregulated markets are not to be trusted, and where negative social and/or economic consequences have arisen, is more pragmatic in its methods of implementing social democratic policies: it believes that there is a need for major structural change, and regulation should interfere with the harsh systematic market agenda, promoting the development of emerging markets and developing nations, assisting in the creation of new ways of directing systematic market outcomes to ensure a more equal distribution of social goods.

Any answer to the global financial crisis must take into account the social costs, because human suffering through market failure is disproportionally affecting the developing countries, as well as the poor in richer countries where the labour markets are being put under increasing pressure. The stability of a workable banking and financial system within the global economy produces a means to an end, not an end in itself. Ultimately, it is ends that matter, ends that are social.

As Quiggin points out, social democracy needs to learn from past mistakes:

> The current period of financial crises began in the late 1990s has demonstrated the falsity of many of the assumptions underlying economic liberalism, and, in particular, of claims about the microeconomic and macroeconomic superiority of free markets. Nevertheless economic liberals were correct in pointing out some of the policy mistakes made under the postwar social democratic settlement. It is important that a resurgent social democracy should avoid repeating those mistakes (Quiggin, 2009:15).

Works Consulted

Etzioni, A. (2001), 'The Third-Way is a triumph', *New Statesman* (1996), Volume 130, Issue 4543, 1–4, http://infotrac.galegroup.com/itw/infomark/550/4/4504 8019w6/purl=rc1_EAIM_0_A76665963&dyn=5!xrn_ 1_0_A76665963?sw_aep=unimelb.

Finn, D. (2002), Interview with Peter Gibilisco, unpublished.

Gibilisco, P. (2004a), 'Global Economic Reform at the Local Level: social aspects of service provision for people with disabilities', Inaugural 3D Conference, Department of Public Health, University of Melbourne, Conference Paper, 1–13.

Gibilisco, P. (2004b), 'Is the Victorian government trying to avoid helping people in need?', *On Line Opinion*, February 16, 1–2, http://www.onlineopinion.com.au/view.asp?article=18 82.

Gibilisco, P. (2008c), 'Universal access to disability services defines our progress', *On Line Opinion*, http://www.onlineopinion.com.au/view.asp?article=82 31.

Gibilisco, P. (2009b), 'Financial crisis, social democracy and social policy', *On the ine Opinion*, October 29, 1–3, http://www.onlineopinion.com.au/view.asp?article=96 07.

Gibilisco, P. (2009c), 'Is the 'Third-Way' the right way?', *On Line Opinion*, July 7, 1–2, http://www.onlineopinion.com.au/view.asp?article=91 01.

Gibilisco, P. (2009d), 'The Third-Way', *Just Policy*, April, Edition 50, 43–49.

Johnson, C. (2002), Interview with Peter Gibilisco, unpublished.

Nursey-Bray, P. (2001), 'What Directions Are Left?', *Left Directions: Is there a Third-Way?* Nursey-Bray, P and Bacchi, C (eds), University of West Australia Press, Crawley, 52–66.

Orchard, L. (1989), 'Public Choice Theory and the Common Good', *Markets, Morals and Public Policy*—Orchard, L. and Dare, R. (eds), The Federation Press, Annandale, pp. 265–281.

Orchard, L. (2002), Interview with Peter Gibilisco, unpublished.

Quiggin, J. (2009), 'An agenda for Social Democracy', *Perspectives*, Whitlam Institute, April 6, 1–16, http://www.whitlam.org/whitlam/images/whitlam_pers pectives_1.pdf.

Russell, M. (2000a), 'The Political Economy of Disablement', *Dollars and Sense*, September, 1–7, http://www.disweb.org/marta/ped.html.

Russell, M. (2001b), 'New Freedom Initiative: Survival of the Fittest "Equality"', Znet Daily Commentaries, 1–5, http://www.zmag.org/sustainers/content/2001-02/23russell.htm.

Russell, M. (2001c), 'What's Wrong with "Charitable Choice"? A Plenty', Znet Daily Commentaries, 1–5, http://www.zmag.org/sustainers/content/2001-03/28russell.htm.

Russell, M. (2002), 'The Social Movement Left Out', Z net: Daily commentaries, 1–5. http://www.zmag.org/sustainers/content/2002-08/31russell.cfm.

Sen, A. (1999), *Development as Freedom*, Anchor Books, New York.

Shorten, B. (2009), 'WA Disability Collective Lecture Series', unpublished, University of Western Australia, June 4, 1–26.

Stretton, H. (1996), Poor Laws of 1834 and 1996, occasional paper, Brotherhood of St Laurence, Fitzroy.

Stretton, H. (2003), Interview with Peter Gibilisco, unpublished.

Tanner, L. (2002), Interview with Peter Gibilisco, unpublished.

The White House—President (2009), 'The Agenda—
Disabilities', 1–2,
http://www.whitehouse.gov/agenda/disabilities.

Wearne, B. (2009), Interview with Peter Gibilisco, unpublished.

CHAPTER 4

Education for People with
Severe Physical Disabilities

Insights into the political economy of education for people with severe physical disabilities

> The politics of the world have shifted from the Keynesian welfare state to the neo-liberal post-welfare state. The current educational policies arise out of the need for governments to retain legitimacy by appearing to be doing something about the increasing economic inequality, to support capital accumulation through the reduction of taxes and the education of workers, and, particularly for neoconservatives in response to the social unrest of the 1960s and 1970s, to regain social control (Hursh, 2005).

Today, one can view with utter contempt the institutionalisation of people with disabilities that was identified with the need for custodial care. This style of dehumanising institutionalisation was brought about during the industrial revolution, where people with disabilities were viewed as those who did not need education but, instead, constant and institutionalised supervision.

During the 19th century, people with disabilities were openly discriminated against, and thereby were excluded from mainstream society. They were automatically regarded as feeble-minded, and as a burden on society. Society's response was to lock them away from public sight, an extreme form of social exclusion (Sen, 1999).

Such historical processes have aided the stereotyping of people with disabilities that still runs strongly throughout 20th century intellectual thought and social practice. The human fear of difference was embraced throughout the 20th century, right from the early years of *laissez-faire* economics and mass production, when the institutionalisation of people with disabilities was considered mandatory. As Jenny Cooper puts it:

> Hitler was in good company; Winston Churchill had stated shortly before that the 'increasingly rapid growth of the feeble-minded classes—constitutes a race danger—the source from which the stream of madness is fed should be cut off and sealed up before

another year has passed'[2]. Among his supporters were D.H. Lawrence, H.G. Wells and Aldous Huxley. Up until 1971, a whole section of the disabled community was still labelled 'ineducable' and even when they were 'brought in' to the education system in 1971, they were still described as 'educationally subnormal'. We grew up hearing these terms, and shocked that our grandparents grew up hearing 'idiot', 'imbecile' and 'feeble-minded.' Is it any wonder we foster low expectations for disabled people in education? (Cooper, 2006:1)

Equality within the broad spectrum of people with disabilities has been called 'the last civil rights movement' but is this based on a hierarchy of stereotypes, which define the inclusiveness of a person with disabilities (Cooper, 2006:4)?

For example, this is from the Master's thesis of Professor Yvonne Singer, who today is an online professor at two American universities, she put her past experiences in these terms: "The investigator, [has cerebral palsy, leaving her a severely physically disabled woman with slurred speech,]

---

[2] British Film Industry (http://bfi.org.uk); *Education on Disability*

personally encountering many hardships involving discrimination" (Singer 2002:1).

Living in a non-institutionalised environment, maintaining high self-efficacy and being well educated did not change how employers viewed her. After earning her Bachelor of Psychology from Monmouth University in 1999, she submitted 100 resumes to various human service organisations and web design positions. As a result, the investigator received a total of 100 rejection letters, requests for money donations, and address labels. Once employers discovered that she was disabled they ignored all her qualifications and refused to interview her (Singer, 2002:31).

In David Hursh's critical reflection, the rise of a global meritocracy within the US, and within most other western countries, has transformed the education system, with the major focus upon degrees, subjects and graduates who, it is a widely held view, it is presumed will assist in increasing economic productivity. Hursh puts it like this:

Creating appropriately skilled and entrepreneurial citizens and workers able to generate new and added economic values will enable nations to be responsive to changing conditions within the international market-place (Hursh, 2003:1).

Such a view is dominant in many societies, typically taken to promote professional degrees, at the expense of the basic BA (Arts) and BSc (Science) degrees. Stretton argues that the quality of life and social inclusiveness of people with disabilities today is significantly affected by the quality, experience and effect of the higher education system, with its increasing influence on future prospects of employment. This could create the makings of a prosperous future for people with disabilities, but instead it is severely restricted by poor education, which follows on to poor professional employment opportunities, which can also worsen social exclusion. Today, in the educational spectrum 'the picture does not look so good anymore. Inclusion is happening, but mainly for those with milder disabilities' (Cooper, 2006:3).

Meanwhile, developments in information and communications technology have fundamentally changed the skills required for a wide range of jobs, and so have influenced the general attitude of societies to the usefulness of education. For example, today it is extremely difficult to get employed in a management position without a degree.

In the fields of technology and communication, appropriate education and skills are conditions that are capable of being developed by most people, including many people with disabilities. This potential will only be achieved with appropriate social policy providing that the means to ensure people with disabilities get a fair chance at entering and proceeding in the higher education system.

The Pensioner Education Supplement

The Liberal–National government attempted to reduce entitlements for students with disabilities in the 2003 budget by not paying the educational supplement over the three-month summer break, in effect cutting the supplement by 25 per cent. The Pensioner Education Supplement (PES) is a meagre education supplement that can be applied for by those on the pension, but the government could see the wisdom of reducing this already small entitlement, even though, presumably, students would be preparing for study over the summer break anyway.

The PES was first introduced under the federally funded Austudy–Abstudy scheme in 1987, and since 1998 it has been funded through Centrelink. The Pensioner Education Supplement was introduced to provide those in receipt of a pension with an incentive to further their education. It offered small financial incentives to be used towards the extra cost of study materials. It is a flat payment of about $30 a week and a once-yearly 'entry into education' payment of about $200 (Devlin, as cited in Gibilisco, 2011).

In 2003, Amanda Vanstone, then Minister for Family and Community Services, stated in the Senate:

> If you take two people who are pensioners—one of whom is not studying and one who is—over the summer break they will be in the same position, because the one who is studying is not attending their university or TAFE course over the summer break and is therefore not in need of the supplement. They will not be without assistance. They will be in the same position as hundreds of thousands of other disability support pensioners who are not undertaking tertiary study (Vanstone, as cited in Gibilisco, 2011).

This is but one example of a prominent politician failing to understand the diverse 'life problems' that are likely to arise from a disability. The practical fulfilment of higher education for people with disabilities can help to alleviate some of these problems. For people with disabilities, higher education can help to lift self-esteem.

This issue, in particular, filled me with rage, and with good reason. From 1993 to 1997, I was a recipient of this meagre supplement. Even though the extra benefit was nowhere near enough, it was something. It helped to keep my head above water, in a learning environment not suited to many people with disabilities. An education expense incurred during my years of study was the substantial cost of the M50 (a vehicle capable of transporting those confined to the wheelchair) taxi fares, particularly when attending the Peninsula Campus of Monash University, because public transport is definitely not suitable to somebody in my condition (Friedreich's ataxia).

During this time I attended classes about three times a week for the 26-week period: a round trip in the taxi cost about $30. While the extraordinary expense was not entirely covered by the PES it did provide some contribution, thereby enabling me to complete my undergraduate studies. In 1997,

I completed a Masters qualifying year at the Clayton campus of Monash University, where, for doing this, I was in receipt of the PES and my taxi costs were about the same.

I decided to speed up the process of getting a degree by taking on summer school. For many people with severe physical disabilities, and despite Vanstone's comments, there is no break from regularity of the day-to-day existence provided by a disability. Cutting out the pittance of additional support we get through the pensioner education supplement further limits the choices of higher education for students with disabilities.

According to Vanstone, by reducing the supplement to pensioners, we would save $39 million in four years. Such savings would reduce the governmental burden of social spending and add to the prospects of a healthy budget surplus. Despite the government's attempt to remove the PES for the summer break, they were not successful, as the bill was unable to gain passage through a hostile Senate; for this particular bill the government failed to gain the support of the Upper House.

The digital revolution

The digital revolution may equip some people with disabilities with the information technology that has the potential, when combined with ongoing political and social struggle, to free our society from the realities of disability.

But, in the digital age 'disability' is also socially constructed through such technology, which in itself can prevent adequate solutions to real social problems for such people. Many cannot afford to become part of this solution. Besides other barriers, the equipment costs are simply beyond the means of those who survive on the disability pension. The digital revolution can create additional barriers for people with disabilities. Commentators regularly speak of a 'digital divide'—a widening of the socioeconomic gap—which, for people with disabilities, is exacerbated even further.

Technology can widen rather than help close these gaps. These gaps are highlighted when the disposable income available through the disability pension is compared with the average disposable income of the able bodied. And so, the digital revolution may be at the forefront of widening the gap between the educational and interrelated disparities of people with disabilities and most of society's other so-called 'normal' members.

People with disabilities need a collective and empathetic approach so as not to add to the social exclusion and impoverishment they already feel with respect to mainstream society. They need to be regarded as more than just the stereotype of people with lesser abilities. They need collective assurances that using technology to develop new skills is not an elusive dream. As a severely physically disabled person, I believed the idea of developing self-esteem through the gaining of a PhD sounded attractive.

However many ideas are often attractive in theory but destructive in practice. The price of computers, for example, can be a big issue for the average disabled pensioner. Some of the costs involved are:

- a working computer with required software

- installation—having a motor-function type of disability stops me from installing my own computer

- connection to the Internet and the persistent monthly bills

- after-sales service and constant purchase of the required computer programs and accessories, printing paper and ink

This takes a large sum of cash from a meagre entitlement such as the disability pension, which is fixed at far less than the needed fortnightly rate, leaving one with little, if any, disposable income for any further computer hardware and software, or upkeep.

Again, this shows the need for continual intervention from government to realise that concepts such as merit are not neutral, but are socially constructed. In this example, my capacity to participate in higher education on the basis of merit was severely constrained by factors such as, for example, the inadequate provision of collective entitlements for people with disabilities, i.e. limited finances.

People with disabilities are also often in situations where the social structures around them are inadequate: the dominant political agenda reinforces this with the theory that fewer entitlements are the much needed spur to create more empowerment. So by reforming social policy with fewer entitlements, which in turn increases the government's budget surplus, they can then justifiably further reduce taxes.

Gerald Goggin and Christopher Newell argue '[n]ew communication and media technologies will also offer some puta-
tive solutions—but these may well be solutions to social
problems masked by the beneficent face of technology'
(2003:153). Many people with disabilities cannot afford to
become part of this solution. Besides other barriers the
equipment costs are simply beyond their means. As they put
it:

> It is not so much the latest add-on, the fastest com-
> puter, or even the more expansive application or uni-
> versal design that will confer the greatest benefit for
> people with disabilities. Rather, we need to recognise
> that in whatever we do we have the opportunity to dis-
> able or enable. We recommend that it is time for soci-
> ety to decide that it wishes to reconnect with people
> with disabilities in the digital future that will be our
> emerging society. This is not so much a technological
> question, as a political one (Goggin and Newell,
> 2003:154).

This divide between the able bodied and people with disabilities is also destined to be further widened by the neoliberal political economic response to globalisation. This market-driven, merit-based, political economic response will only further add to the impoverishment and social exclusion of most people with disabilities.

Globalisation and the knowledge society

Orchard explains that globalisation is not just an economic process, but also involves technological and cultural processes. Proponents of the third-way view the technological and cultural visions as a global expression of the knowledge society. For example, the third-way acknowledges the improvements in ideas that are available in different cultures, as information concerning much needed ideas. These are made more readily available and readable through technological improvements to communication, such as the timely transference of information via the Internet.

The writings of former ALP leader Mark Latham, for example, argue that the information age and globalisation are tailor made for progressive politics of the third-way kind. Therefore, the third-way, according to Latham, is the best way to deliver these opportunities to all who may benefit from such processes. It is a process that allows many more of society's members to engage constructively in a globalised society, generating wealth and prosperity by harnessing the brain-power, or knowledge, of individuals.

The major force, knowledge capitalism, driving the new world economy is as pervasive and powerful as financial capitalism, but as yet less materially recognised. It is a force that generates new ideas and turns them into products and services. In the new economy, when you buy products today, you primarily pay for the intelligence ingrained in their software and technological format.

Knowledge-based resources are the goal for the political economy of the 21st century. The creation and dispersion of knowledge in society has the potential to achieve the fundamental aim of balancing the difficulties of the markets against those related problems in the community. In this regard, the goals of becoming a knowledge-driven society may also be viewed as radical and emancipatory.

Many believe that the knowledge society will incorporate far reaching implications that include improving the ways companies are owned, managed and organised. Such improvements are, in part, made possible through various global ventures to benchmark best practice. A knowledge society can also help in the acknowledgement of rewards, and the distribution of talent, creativity and the contribution of actions. This has the capability of highlighting educational factors, such as modes of learning that are research organised through the Internet and other means.

Public investment in education is the best way to ensure the constant rebuilding of social capital. It is through the processes of education that we are better able to understand the human importance of social capital. By providing a knowledge society the choice between the economics of capitalism and community is avoided, as a highly skilled population will enjoy the benefits of both.

Education generates a more efficient economy, and a more cohesive and trusting society. Global economic trends have helped more people than ever before to move out of poverty by creating new ways of creating social capital and by allowing access to alternative forms of finance.

The three major priorities that will improve the integrity, cohesiveness and wellbeing of a globally integrated society are education, entrepreneurship and reward for effort. A knowledge nation is capable of a more effective understanding of political change, influenced in many ways through a surge in technologies.

The technological surge has bought about changes in communication and trade that have increased the demand for a globally structured market economy. This in turn places more emphasis on compliance with global markets, which enforces a reduced emphasis on the role of the state to satisfy society's economic and social demands. Botsman argues that a knowledge society is more capable of providing opportunities for individual success, and that global companies today have the capacity to construct products anywhere, and sell them everywhere, radically changing the political economy of western and other nations.

Others, in contrast, disagree, arguing that the knowledge economy is structured on the conservative political provision of freedom and competition. In addition, equality of opportunity is also regarded as an economic necessity, which, in effect, prioritises and rewards the strategy of economic efficiency over social integrity. The knowledge economy can be

identified with the competitive skills of the workforce, allowing today's concept of meritocracy to be more associated
with the individualised policies of neoliberalism and the
third-way.

The dominant political approach

The market logic today changes citizens into clients. This ap-
plies particularly in the arena of education, acknowledging
the important role that the education sector has in the global
pursuit of economic productivity. Our productivity and contribution to the country's economy is now, more than ever, a
matter for the state. The third-way, in practice, harnesses the
globally based politics of meritocracy that view individual
merit as a basis for approval. For many people in society, it is
culturally accepted that people with disabilities have less
ability to develop merit, thereby confirming the bias in the
social construction of the concept of merit itself.

Despite this, third-way sympathisers like Latham and Clinton
endorsed the strategy of less entitlement and more empowerment for welfare recipients, including those with disabilities.

The key to the social inclusion of people with disabilities is their ability to gain employment and thereby to function more fully as members of society. Work placement and recruitment depend, in turn, on the ability to meet the procedural requirements of the necessary education and training needs.

The global marketplace has brought about a paradigm shift. This paradigm is structured upon continual innovation, reform, restructuring and benchmarking government and non-government authorities. Some believe that the third-way will enhance society in the global world, using global techniques built into a knowledge economy. This in turn will enhance education and training as core elements for the new world. An educated society could be the key to the social harmony of society.

Thus, the third-way has proactive concerns about an educated society, believing that society as a whole will benefit if most of its people are educated. For example, the breakdown of dominant stereotypes of people with disabilities must come through education. However, problems again arise when this concern is connected to a more general third-way philosophy

of reducing state intervention. Given the short-term impera-
tives of business in capitalist societies to make profits, the
expectation that such businesses freely invest in higher education for people with disabilities is somewhat misplaced and
probably idealistic.

Disability advocacy:
why does it elude those most in need?

When looking to the National Disability Advocacy Program
(NDAP), a new updated site, many people with high-support
needs will believe there is plenty left to be achieved in disability advocacy (FAHCSIA, 2012). Still, advocates in the
disability sector are in general unaware of what is holding up
the implementation of processes that would advance such inclusion.

The NDAP has as its main objective the provision of assistance to people with disabilities in order that communities
become inclusive of people with such human differences in
an ongoing recognition of their rights. These aspirations have
been stated under its aims and objectives:

- Provide appropriate and timely advocacy to people with disability that addresses instances of abuse, discrimination and neglect.

- Inform people with disability about their rights and responsibilities, and support them where possible in making informed decisions about issues that impact on their lives.

- Contribute to raising community awareness of disability issues.

- Contribute to government policy, service and program development (FAHCSIA, 2012).

However, there is considerable unmet need in advocacy for people with high-support needs. If this lack is recognised, and measures taken to provide adequate advocacy, it will give them their own voice—even if their abilities to communicate are significantly impaired through disability. I number myself among these people. The last time I publicly drew attention to the number of such people in our community was when I was speaking for the Coalition of Disability Rights during the 2006 Victorian state election campaign (Coalition for Disability Rights, 2006).

In 2003, according to the Australian Bureau of Statistics there were just over 300 000 people with high-support needs in Victoria (Coalition for Disability Rights, 2006). And there are many people with such needs who should, and probably would, avail themselves of high-support services if there were a more powerful advocacy on their behalf. No doubt we need a better understanding about the best way to advocate our needs, but we also need to avail ourselves of the skills that are offered by advocates of people with high-support needs. Better understanding all around would undoubtedly increase demands and also open up the life possibilities for all concerned.

Consider the fact that many people with high-support needs are not able to access such advocacy services due to a lack of awareness and decreased capabilities that result from an inability to pick up the phone and make initial contact. In other words, they have a lack of awareness of the kind of downward spiral that becomes commonplace to many of those with high-support needs.

This is further noted by the failure of the Department of

Families, Housing, Community Services and Indigenous Affairs Internet home page (FAHCSIA, 2012). Although this page has been recently updated, it still can be difficult to navigate through for many people with communication impairments and high-support needs. At a first glance, it is difficult to find easy English web pages to explain the NDAP. What I'm trying to point out is that we need a policy that will help deliver an upward spiral.

Jenny Cooper reports in 'Inclusion our destiny?':

> Looking at worldwide trends, the pattern in countries with supposedly the most progressive records of inclusion is that the most severely disabled get left behind, i.e. an even smaller minority even more segregated (Cooper, 2006).

At one stage my support worker gave advice to another severely disabled client who required an advocate, and who was unaware such specific services existed. Once he had made that initial contact to an advocate they were able to assist him appropriately. I know of this case because my support worker acted as 'interim advocate' to link this fellow with the necessary form of advocacy.

That's the link I'm trying to put my finger on here.

So it is not only a matter of there being a need for an increase in funding. There is also a vital need for an **increase in awareness** within the disability sector, especially about what needs to be funded to help the advocacy process of people with high-support needs. Individual advocacy is needed to enhance the lives of people with high-support needs by advocating for support and empowerment.

Jenny Cooper also believes that society has not yet fully acknowledged that people with severe disabilities have feelings and the right to dignity. The point is that people only act if they believe it is bad enough. There is a need to tolerate diversity and a need to live alongside those with high-support needs.

For example, a person with a severe disability, such as myself, might search the Internet to find an applicable advocate via the social media, such as on Facebook and or similar platforms. Because some people cannot communicate via traditional methods such media raise the hope that new levels of society-wide awareness can be achieved.

Living with a severe and progressive disability

It is probable that everyone will get an itch somewhere, sooner or later. And so, when you get an itch, you do what comes naturally—you scratch it! It is a simple process that itches are made to feel better when scratched. Or so it seems. But what if you can't scratch? I mean, what if you can't scratch where it itches because you have nothing to scratch it with? It may be an itch that is underneath your plaster cast that is in place to help with the healing of your broken knee-cap. What if the itch can't be localised? What then? It is not such a simple problem.

I happen to know a lot about the problem of scratching itches from a rather unique perspective. How? Because I have a neurotransmitter dysfunction that simply won't allow me to reach wherever it itches. So I have learnt to cope, to block out the irritation. I have to admit that it is, indeed, a luxury when I am fortunate enough to have a very empathetic support worker who can help me by scratching my back or my ear, but I won't bore you with all the details of my relief because I have only raised this with another purpose in mind, a purpose I might add that might help our society understand the itches people like myself have to deal with. Living with a degenerative disease has broadened my thoughts concerning disablement and allowed me to focus on the need for empathetic behaviour from those directly related to disability. In 1981, I was 19. That was the year of the first United Nations International Year for Disabled People. You'd have to say that my life, with the progression of Friedreich's ataxia since then, has tracked the development of public policy that has, in significant ways, taken seriously the problems that people with disabilities have to continually and progressively confront. In this sense, mainstream society has begun to acknowledge disablement as a serious itch that needs to be carefully scratched with appropriate care, tools and resources that are outlined in socially just policies. And so there are policies, legislation, a wider social commitment, education and programs now in place that show, in this country, that we have a significant society-wide compassion to assist those in great need. But, yet the itch is still not getting appropriately scratched!

Yes, we need ramps and railings that lead into public buildings. But, there needs to be something more. Let me tell you that I have received much, for which I am very grateful. And have come such a long way with so many people to thank. I often wonder, how can someone like me have got this far? And with a disease that has made a greater impact over my body as time passes. I am now 52 and my care needs increase almost by the day. Yet despite this I have completed a study tour in Hawaii, visiting the University of Hawaii's Centre for Disability Studies. My social enquiry in the US focused on how many people with severe disabilities yearn for, and are capable of performing, most human activities—with assistance from a support worker.

It was 1984 when I started my development in higher education, but this year reminds us of something else, doesn't it? Since then, my life has been not unlike the problematic world that George Orwell describes. It is especially relevant to people like myself who are really very grateful for all the special consideration, no matter how insignificant, equal opportunities and affirmative action we have received over the years.

But why is it problematic? It is problematic in an Orwellian sense because we know that if we raise a voice in criticism, even if we are trying to be constructive, we put ourselves in an exposed situation. After having travelled so far, with so much kind assistance, it can too easily sound like we can never be satisfied and can never get enough freebies.

It's as if after graduating with my PhD, and then in 2007 when I was presented with the Emerging Disability Leader of the Year award, I developed a new itch, but just didn't know where, so it couldn't be scratched. My PhD thesis, my academic journal articles and my *On Line Opinion* pieces were all being applauded but, somehow, the major issue I was trying to discuss was being ignored.

I think public policies towards people with disabilities, and in particular severely disabled or progressively disabled, have ignored some important factors to the detriment of our society. I know I sound like a broken record by offering my analysis over and over again, but I also feel that our society cannot be, or become, the compassionate solidarity it claims for itself if it doesn't hear what I am trying to say. I have a sense of obligation here to speak out. It's not just for me, although I am painfully aware of its application to myself and to my own situation.

The point is this: for some of us the special consideration, equal opportunity and affirmative action, designed to get people with disabilities into the mainstream, paradoxically brings us to a more exposed and needy situation. This cannot be addressed without more special consideration, further and ongoing application of equal opportunities after training is completed, and further affirmative action once we have obtained our qualifications. It is a simple point that can be readily illustrated.

This illustration of policy dynamism is based on the approach I have identified as pragmatic social democracy, advocated by Hugh Stretton and many others, in my doctoral dissertation. Once a person with a severe disability, at TAFE for example, receives a diploma then society's responsibility to that person is not somehow fulfilled, because at that point the obligations have actually increased. The person may need special support to attend interviews, and when that person is offered and accepts a position of employment it may be necessary for technical and other assistance.

I could repeat this point for each of the steps I have made through my own higher education: TAFE Diploma, Bachelor of Business, Bachelor of Arts, Master of Arts, and Doctorate of Philosophy. There are other facets to keep in mind as well.

Somehow we need to find a way to view and support people with a disability using proactive methods of equal opportunity; rather than focusing on the medical model's view of a sympathetic approach. People with severe disabilities need an empathetic approach aligned to the social model. My assertion is that society's responsibility increases in specific ways oriented to professional commitment and involvement once the student with a severe disability graduates.

As my own needs, and possibly those of others, have increased or are increasing, support should not only be seen in educational terms. The dynamic of increasing support reflected in policy should also seek to meet the increased needs that the policy, at an earlier point, has also helped to bring about. There are also increased needs of those who support, as well as the increasing needs of the person with a disability.

For a TAFE graduate like myself, I was faced with a daunting prospect. I had a wonderful Technical and Further Education (TAFE) experience, which confirmed me as a mature-age student, and I was no different in some ways from any other TAFE graduate: 'What next?' we asked. Leaving TAFE for all of us in that year was a life-changing experience, but life moves on.

Life moves on. That is the irony that is central to my attempt to point to the dynamic at work here. But the paradox is that not all of us, and not all people with disabilities, have to deal with a progressive disease. To apply for a job in an accountancy firm after my graduation from TAFE would have been to ask the prospective employer to initiate a general policy change that we, as a society, were only just beginning to think about, let alone implement.

The political consideration of equal opportunity and affirmative action was still at an early stage. So, as I look back on it now, it is no wonder that I was attracted to the higher education field, which proved to be more advanced, and hence more hospitable to me with my particular needs, than most other areas. I am the beneficiary of higher education that has been required to make room for people with disabilities. But then, it seems that higher education was also being reorientated to make it compatible with job training for a post-industrial society. In such an environment, as Marta Russell has pointed out, a university degree becomes the evidence that society has met its obligations to help people with disabilities compete. Equal opportunity was not always matched with appropriate affirmative action.

In this respect, I would suggest that affirmative action needs to be taken to a new level. And perhaps this new level cannot be reached without recognising the ongoing obligation that a degree-granting institution has to its graduates.

Understanding mutual obligation from the institution to its highly qualified graduates is downplayed—if not lost entirely. In my own case, a university that takes a qualified postgraduate student with Friedrich's ataxia into its PhD programs should not view itself as giving a sympathetic expression according to the biomedical model's agenda, which has the unfortunate ability of institutionalising stereotypes via disability policy. That is, I am sorry to say, the predominant way in which Australian higher education under third-way and neoliberal policies tends to view such achievements.

That's the itch I have wanted to scratch. We need universities that will recognise their institutional mutual obligation is not transacted merely by granting degrees, and then every year thereafter sending out brochures inviting its highly qualified alumni to give generously to the university's noble cause.

In my case, I am forced to ask: how is it that the university has not required me to give back by doing post-doctoral research and to be part of its ongoing research effort? How is it that it can take on a candidate without expecting to maintain its responsibility to provide ongoing support after graduation?

Note my point is not to ask that my work be judged before I do it. I am referring here to the lack of effort or empathy that seems to come from the side of those administrating higher education institutions in Australia. Writing pieces for media outlets such as *On Line Opinion*, or developing my own blog, are indeed satisfying experiences and I would not want them to be taken away. But such personal satisfaction as getting a paper published is not the main game. What I am concerned about is the development of genuine policy for the severely disabled, and, in particular, policies that will seek to meet needs that arise from progressive disability.

Works Consulted

Botsman, P. (2002), Interview with Peter Gibilisco, unpublished.

Coalition for Disability Rights (2006), Broad Coalition Tells Politicians: 'Disability Counts'. Disability News: Infoxchange Australia;
http://www.disabilitynews.infoxchange.net.au/news/detail.chtml?filename_num=94350.

Cooper, J (2006). Inclusion our destiny? Education for tomorrow, 88,
http://www.educationfortomorrow.org.uk/2006/88inclusion.html.

FAHCSIA, (2012), National Disability Advocacy Program. The Department of Families, Housing, Community Services and Indigenous Affairs. The Australian Government. Canberra; http://www.fahcsia.gov.au/about-fahcsia/overview.

Gibilisco, P. (2007a), 'Barriers to study for the disabled', *On Line Opinion*, February 6, 1–2, http://www.onlineopinion.com.au/view.asp?article=5411.

Gibilisco, P. (2008b), 'Itches and Scratches—living with disability', *On Line Opinion* , March 19, 1–3, http://www.onlineopinion.com.au/view.asp?article=7127.

Gibilisco, P. (2011d), 'Disability advocacy: why does it elude those most in need, *On Line Opinion*, June 6, 1–2, http://www.onlineopinion.com.au/view.asp?article=12135.

Gibilisco, P. (2011g), Politics, Disability and Social Inclusion: People with different abilities in the 21st Century, VDM Verlag, Saarbrücken.

Goggin, G. and Newell, C. (2003), Digital Disability: The social construction of disability in new media, Rowman and Littlefeild Publishers Incorporated, Oxford.

Hursh, D. (2003), 'Neoliberalism and schooling in the U.S, 'How state and federal government education policies perpetuate inequality', *Journal for Critical Education Policy*, Volume 1, Number 2, downloaded to Word, pp. 1–17, http://www.jceps.com/index.php?pageID=article&articleID=12.

Hursh, D. (2005). Neo-liberalism, markets and accountability: Transforming education and undermining democracy in the United States and England. *Policy Futures in Education,* 3:1.

Orchard, L. (1989), 'Public Choice Theory and the Common Good', *Markets, Morals and Public Policy*, Orchard, L. and Dare, R. (eds), The Federation Press, Annandale, pp. 265–281.

CHAPTER 5

Employment and its Economic and Social Empowerment of People with Disabilities

> Society still perceives disability as a medical matter. That is, society associates disability with physiological, anatomical, or mental 'defects' and holds these conditions responsible for the disabled person's lack of full participation in the economic life of our society, rather than viewing their exclusion for what it is—a matter of hard constructed socio-economic relations that impose isolation (and poverty) upon disabled people. This medicalization of disability places the focus on curing the so-called abnormality—the blindness, mobility impairment, deafness, mental or developmental condition—rather than constructing work environments where one can function with such impairments (Russell, 2000b:1).

Insights into the political economy of employment for people with disabilities

People with disabilities have a lower labour-force participation rate than people without disabilities. During the years between 1998 and 2003 the employment rate for people with disabilities was constantly 30 per cent lower for males and 22–25 per cent lower for females when compared to the rates of people without disabilities (AIHW, 2008:22).

However, when we take into account the participation rate for people with severe or profound limitations the levels of unemployment were lower again than for people with minor disabilities. Even acknowledging an increased rate of participation for people with minor disabilities, corresponding with recent strong growth in the labour market, there is still no improvement in employment rates for people with severe or profound limitations, only a further decline. This low employment rate is also a major contributor to the low levels of household income, and thus is a major cause of the high rate of poverty among people with disabilities.

So, how does employment affect the lives of people with disabilities? Employment can have a range of benefits for all, especially those in minority groups who have been socially marginalised and who have often been denied access to employment. Employing people with disabilities can have both economic benefits and can also improve the skill levels of people with disabilities and thereby integrate them into mainstream society. Therefore, public and private policies should be aimed at encouraging the employment of all people with disabilities (AIHW, 2008:22).

The lack of opportunity to provide a satisfactory quality of life for themselves and their families experienced by many people with disabilities is due to their socially reduced capacity to earn income. This is the outstanding feature of their, as yet unfulfilled, employment capability (Sen, 1999). This reduction in employment capability is identified by Russell as being due to stereotypical beliefs held by employers and society at large. For example, it is generally believed that employment of people with disabilities will mean lower productivity, reducing the profit cycles of companies in the private sector. Many forms of prejudice and discrimination are known to exist, such as insinuations that people with physical disabilities are also intellectually disabled, or vice versa. These stereotypes serve to exclude many people with disabilities from paid employment.

Russell argues that employers have justified high unemployment among people with disabilities by claiming that they are unable to keep pace with the demands of the workplace.

The employment problem for people with disabilities is also driven by the dominance of the biomedical model, which identifies disability as an individual problem, rather than the result of economic, political, cultural and social factors.

In health care, the biomedical model of health and illness has systematically dominated with disability being primarily viewed within the medical diagnosis of physiological, ana-tomical, or mental defects (Russell, 2001a:1–3). This model is then captured in legislation, with United States Social Se-curity law, defining 'disabled' as medically unable to engage in work activity (Berkowitz cited in Russell, 2001a:2).

This approach identifies people with disabilities as biologi-cally inferior, which then becomes a means of social control that relegates them from full participation in social and eco-nomic life. This biomedical approach focuses on curing the medical impairment, as opposed to assistance in all areas, particularly in areas where medicine has little to offer. At the same time, it functions according to the belief that people with disabilities are unable to participate fully in society until their abnormality is cured. In other words, the focus of the biomedical model in the context of disability and employment is on fixing the individual, rather than transforming the workplace.

Many forms of social exclusion related to disability are emerging from the value system and policy prescriptions of a market-driven economy. The resultant political economy depends upon the private sector; when the market is driven in this way the problems faced by people with disabilities increase and are exacerbated by prejudicial or discriminatory attitudes. The market-driven system must put profits before people, and so the stigmas and disutilities that are already associated with the employment of people with disabilities are reinforced; employers assume that they will have lowered productivity if they employ workers with disabilities. In the context of the US, Russell argues:

> Despite a growing economy and a 29-year low official unemployment rate, potential workers with disabilities remain chronically unemployed. Nine years after the passage of the *Americans with Disabilities Act* (ADA), national employment surveys show no real statistical

gain in employment for people with disabilities, rather, the unemployment rate remains at 70 per cent, with only three out of ten working full or part-time compared to eight out of ten of those without disabilities—a gap of fifty percentage points (Russell, 1999b:1).

Russell identifies the third-way economically with neoliberalism.

Russell (2003c:6) argues that '[n]eo-classical supply and demand models posit that the labour market will equalize pay and employment differentials.' From this neoclassical viewpoint, the market pay inequalities are little more than the natural result of the spread of information technologies, which makes use of marketable skills. This provides higher pay and status for educated people with market-orientated merit, while those without such training fall behind. And so we see the rise of meritocracy in the global competitive workplace.

Russell identifies the market-driven understanding of meritocracy as one that serves as a self-regulating system for wages, prices and production, as a system of individual merit in the workplace that is capable of giving a thriving business its competitive edge.

Market-driven economic theories are echoed by the government policies, which become a key device for measuring people's merits. He argues that third-way provisions for meritocracy are capable of providing for equal opportunity in the workforce. However, policies that enable people with disabilities to engage in paid employment will improve, rather than reduce equality overall.

Russell argues that market-driven beliefs 'challenge the notion that differences in human capital, quality of education, and years of work experience can adequately explain the wage differentials and employment patterns that remain prominent in the economy.' This returns us to the global vision of a merit-based workforce developed by a meritocracy, which creates an unjust employment paradox for many people with disabilities. For example, there are the stereotypical misjudgements concerning the ability of many people with disabilities to fulfil the requirements of employment, such as the belief that most people with disabilities are feeble minded. Many of these stigmas and disutilities are perpetu ated jointly by the meritocratic ideology of neoliberal capitalism.

Identifying some of the obstacles to employment for people with disabilities

The stigma concerning the employment of people with disabilities is encouraged by the already high rates of unemployment among such workers, based on assumptions that they are not as productive compared with able-bodied employees. Such stereotypes are a compound of other various prejudices as well, such as, for example, that people with disabilities have a higher turnover rate, are a safety risk, are too costly to employ, and are too demanding. They would also, likely, be an embarrassment to the organisation, and would not fit in to the organisation's culture. In other words, people with disabilities are believed to be unable to perform at the same cognitive or physical level as the non-disabled worker.

It is the institutional practices supported by such beliefs that create a situation in Australia where, in 1993, the unemployment rate of 22 per cent for people with disabilities was more than double the unemployment rate for the able-bodied population. In 2003, the problem had worsened (see Table 1)

(*Human Rights and Equal Opportunity Commission,* 2005:2).

Unemployment rate for people with disabilities in Australia, 1993–2009

	People with disabilities %			
	1993	**1998**	**2003**	**2009**
Labour-force participation rate	54.9	53.2	53.2	58.2
Unemploy-ment rate	17.8	11.5	8.6	7.8

	People without disabilities %			
	1993	**1998**	**2003**	**2009**
Labour-force participation rate	76.9	80.1	80.6	72.6
Unemploy- ment rate	12.0	7.8	5.0	5.1

Source: ABS, 2003, 26; Productivity Commission, Volume 2: Appendices, A.2. Persons aged 15–64

The labour-force participation rate is the comparative numbers of people with disabilities and people without disabilities active in the labour market. The unemployment rate is the comparative statistics on people with disabilities and people without disabilities without paid employment, but who are actively seeking employment.

This table shows that there are fewer people with disabilities who participate in the workforce than those without disabilities. In 2003, 53.2 per cent of people with disabilities participated in the labour force, in comparison to 80.6 per cent of those without a disability.

> Over the sixteen years from 1993 to 2009, the unemployment rate for 15–64 year olds with disability decreased from 17.8% to 7.8%, in line with the similar decline in unemployment for those with no disability (from 12.0% in 1993 to 5.1% in 2009). However, the unemployment rate for people with disability continued to be significantly higher than for those without disability in 2009 (ABS, 2012).

Also notable from Table 1 is that, between 1993 and 2003, for people without disabilities the labour-force participation rate has increased and the unemployment rate has decreased, while for people with disabilities the labour-force participation rate has decreased, but so also has the unemployment rate. As these figures are based on people who are either active in the labour market, or who are actively seeking to be in the labour market, the figures suggest that many people with disabilities have withdrawn from seeking entry into the labour market. In terms of the role of paid employment in promoting social inclusion, this is clearly not a desirable outcome for people with disabilities, or for society as a whole.

The lower labour-force participation rate in combination with a higher unemployment rate for people with disabilities, compared to people without disabilities, is simply a confirmation that people with disabilities are less likely to be employed. In 1993, a person with a disability was 22 per cent less likely than a person without a disability to be in employment; in 1998 this figure was 26.9 per cent less likely to be employed; and in 2003 the difference had increased to 27.4 (Human Rights and Equal Opportunity Commission, 2005:3). As Russell notes, the labour-force participation problem for people with disabilities around the world is not improving.

Empathy, not sympathy, helps inclusiveness

Of late, my severely progressive disability, Friedreich's ataxia, has maintained its advance on my body. This is, I guess, what I have always expected. But for all that, it is a practical and theoretical fact that the near-end results of this disease are simply beyond the reality of most people.

Many intelligent people who know of me, but have no idea

of my determination, are caught in an intellectual 'Catch 22' situation. That is, how can a person with such a severe progressive disability achieve so much? Their taken-for-granted view of life, of success, of achievement, is somehow challenged because disability is equated with a lack of ability to achieve! How then are 'normal' people ever going to achieve insight that this just isn't so? It just doesn't have to be! In some ways it reminds me that my own views on achievement had to be changed, too. We are led to believe that the 'norms' that prevail in the US, are 'progressive', and so we would expect that those who are in positions of political and societal dominance, who make the claim that they are in support of 'inclusion for all', would believe that such a study as mine would be relevant to contemporary political discourse, and that disability should also be depicted in conventional historical accounts. But that kind of 'progressive' determination is somewhat too abstract and too conservative to encompass some of the infinite progressive changes that are at work in society to make social inclusiveness a reality.

This shift to move people with disabilities from the margins to the mainstream of society, maintains a close correlation with social inclusiveness and the need to fit in with their peers. Thus, the word disability in the past has not been synonymous with fashion or sex appeal. But Bob Dylan's song of the 1960s is still relevant—the times they are *indeed* a changin'.

Such progressive achievements may put a new spin on the stigmas and disutilities that encompass the lives of many people with a severely progressive disability like mine. Please, believe me, there are so many people who feel condemned by such negative stereotypes.

This brings me to the subject of disability rights, and prompts me to ponder these at a deeper level.

Jenny Cooper in her article 'Inclusion our destiny' argues that the human race has an historical and monumental obsession with the idea that the 'body beautiful' can only be portrayed by perfection. Such a portrayal, therefore, does not have a great track record of 'including' people with disabilities (Cooper, 2006).

But many will say this has all been tried before—integration, mainstreaming, normalisation. Is there anything left to say about inclusion? Maybe the time is not for loudly making nice-sounding policy statements, but there's still plenty left to be done and nobody seems quite sure why there is a delay in doing it. Is it bureaucrats not towing their 'party line'? The economy? Fear, perhaps? Fate? Or does the idea of social inclusion or disability rights act as a handy tool for government in the creation of social dilemmas?

What is the reality and what is the rhetoric? What I am trying to say is that the vision for change appears to be there but not the active commitment.

How is this to be achieved for everybody with disabilities? There are infinite forms of disability with infinite actions, which have been stereotyped in comical and other demeaning ways, basically due to a lack of education and an inability, or more likely, an unwillingness, to enforce anti-discrimination laws.

Further to this, Cooper argues that a primary example of this apathy to overcome stereotypes is particularly evident when it comes to people with severe disabilities (Cooper, 2006). When the importance of treating *all* people *equally* is acknowledged, then the broad spectrum of people with disabilities confronts such good intentions; this is 'the last human rights movement.'

But is this label not based on a hierarchy of stereotypes? Does it not define the inclusiveness of a person with disabilities as the final frontier, and therefore suggest that it is the most difficult?

I'm not so sure. When the apparently impressive statistics concerning inclusion worldwide are analysed carefully, a closer look at the figures for the inclusion of those with severe disabilities, including speech impairments, will tell us that our record around the globe is not as good as we'd like to think it is. The statistics simply indicate a serious lack of attention to those with severe bodily disabilities. Inclusion is happening, but mainly for those with milder disabilities.

And so, how do government initiatives and practices in education improve the prospects for inclusion of people with severe disabilities? For the time being there is an increase in the numbers of people with severe disabilities entering mainstream education. Statistics confirm that the number of students with a severe disability who attend mainstream education has increased fourfold since the 1980s. But perhaps public policy is in danger of leaving people with disabilities behind. This is because the growth in participation rates in education has not been matched by an increase in employment.

Legal actions against discrimination for people with disabilities

People with disabilities may use legal rights against discrimination. The Multiple Sclerosis Society of Australia argues that people with disabilities are protected by State and Commonwealth discrimination laws in a number of areas of life, including employment. Protection against discrimination is given under the Federal *Disability Discrimination Act 1992* (DDA) (Australia), which covers a range of activities such as 'direct' and 'indirect' discrimination on an 'Australia-wide basis'. Legal Aid, Victoria, defines these forms of discrimination in the following way:

> Direct discrimination is when someone treats you less favourably, or proposes to treat you less favourably, than they would treat someone else in similar circumstances, who does not have a disability.
>
> Indirect discrimination is when you are expected to meet some sort of criteria that you cannot meet be-

cause of your disability, but which people without your disability probably would be able to meet (Legal Aid, Victoria, 2003: 4–5).

States and Territories each have an *Equal Opportunity Act* and a complaints process that cover similar areas (Legal Aid, Victoria, 2003). The Victorian Act more formally states,

The employee needs to show the meeting of genuine and reasonable actions for employment (Human Rights and Equal Opportunity Commission, Australia).

As Legal Aid, Victoria, states:

For example, an important part of a telephonist's job is to be able to communicate by telephone. But it is not inherent or genuine and reasonable requirement to hold the telephone in the hand ... However, it probably is an inherent or genuine and reasonable requirement of a painter's job to be able to climb ladders and carry paint tins (Legal Aid, Victoria, 2003: 10).

According to Legal Aid, Victoria, and the Human Rights and Equal Opportunity Commission, Australia, the employer has the responsibility of telling job applicants the essential requirements of the work. Whether the particular duties of the job stated by the employer are inherent, or genuine and reasonable, can only be determined on a case-by-case basis. To explore this in more detail, we can consider two specific legal cases. Legal Aid, Victoria, describes a case of direct discrimination *Scott and Bernadette Finney v The Hills Grammar School* [1999] HREOC 14 [July 20, 1999]; and a case of indirect discrimination, *Byham v Preston City Council* [1991] EOC: 92–377. These are represented below in some detail, as they provide insights into the circumstances in which discrimination may arise at law.

Direct discrimination

The parents of a 4½ year-old girl with spina bifida applied to enrol their daughter in the local school. With the application they gave details of her disability and particular needs. They later met the registrar to give him more information about their daughter and her disability.

Some months after the interview, the registrar wrote to the parents to say that the school did not have the appropriate resources to look after their daughter in the manner that she required, and in a way that was suitable for her. The parents complained to the Human Rights and Equal Opportunity Commission (HREOC), claiming that the school had directly discriminated against their daughter.

Decision

The commission agreed that, by refusing the girl's enrolment because of her disability, the school was treating her less favourably than it would treat a child without spina bifida. The Federal Court confirmed that the school had directly discriminated against her.

Indirect discrimination

A man, who regularly attended council meetings, used elbow crutches because of a disability. The council refused to install a lift to the first floor of the council building, hence, he had no means of access other than the stairs. The council intended to relocate the municipal offices at some time in the future. They had made available a person to assist anybody wishing to use the stairs. The man complained to the Equal Opportunity Commission about this indirect discrimination.

Decision

The commission said the requirement to use the stairs was not reasonable in the circumstances, taking into consideration the following:

- Cost of installation of the lift was approximately $150,000.

- The resources of the council were great enough to meet the cost of installing the lift.

- Without the lift, the complainant was unable to reach the first floor independently. A substantial number of other people (such as people using wheelchairs or mothers with prams) would not be able to reach the first floor via the steps.

- The premises is a public building substantially maintained by public money.

- Ratepayers have a right to attend council meetings. (Legal Aid, Victoria, 2003:4,6).

Such actions of discrimination perpetrated against people with disabilities, if accepted into due process, may be legally awarded a just form of compensation under the *Disability Discrimination Act* (1992). Legal action, if it can be properly enforced, can diminish stigmas and disutilities of people with disabilities that impose unjustly on their chances in life. However, Russell argues that this will rarely be properly sanctioned in a competitive market-driven political economy, one that ranks profits ahead of people's welfare. For example, such discriminatory practices can be legally enforced by the hardship rule, which is where the party not in compliance with the *Disability Discrimination Act* can legally claim that they have insufficient funds to remedy the situation. That is illustrated in the US by Russell who puts it like this:

> Ironically, Planet Hollywood, one of the sponsors of the 1995 MDA telethon, was not accessible to those it purported to 'help'. It was willing to raise money to 'help the cripples' but the owners are not willing to take our civil rights seriously. How could the owners—which include Sylvester Stallone, Demi Moore, Bruce Willis and Arnold Schwarzenegger—claim an 'undue hardship' from the ADA [*America Disabilities Act*] accessibility regulations; how could they claim to

be unable to afford to build a ramp over three steps (Russell, 1998c:88)?

This is, of course, extremely relevant to Australia. Russell points out that with today's emphasis on a competitive market, public institutions and profit-seeking firms may put the need for profits above the need to enforce civil rights.

The *Disability Discrimination Act*'s effect on employment of people with disabilities is limited by the hardship clause. This clause allows employers to seek a competitive economic edge, rather than seek to update their current workplace to comply with civil rights legislation. Russell explains it in an American context, which again is relevant to Australia:

> Disabled persons are often isolated and excluded from full participation in work life because from a business perspective, the hiring or retaining of a disabled employee represents nonstandard additional costs when calculated against a company's bottom line (Russell, 2000a:2–3).

Affirmative action for people with disabilities

Affirmative action is a political policy approach that allows for positive steps to be taken to promote equal employment opportunity for socially defined groups who have been sub-jected to structural discrimination, according to factors such as gender, disability, age, and race (Bacchi, 1990, 1996). Af-firmative action legislation stipulates that active steps be taken to promote equal opportunity in a more proactive way than anti-discrimination legislation, which seeks to eliminate unequal treatment as experienced by individuals. The goal of affirmative action is to eliminate disadvantages for which the sufferers cannot legitimately be held responsible. Affirmative action programs seek to hold societies accountable for struc-tural discrimination on socially defined groups, by requiring employers to take active steps to provide equal employment opportunities for groups that suffer from discrimination in employment (Bacchi, 1990; and President Obama's 'Disabil-ity Agenda' *White House—President,* 2009:1).

Stilwell and other advocates of affirmative action argue that it is about more than just a redistribution of income, it is about life chances. People with disabilities, in many cases because of unjustified stereotypes, are often excluded from these life chances. Legally enforceable affirmative action for people with disabilities can mandate that positions be filled by a certain percentage of prospective employees with disabilities.

Russell believes that affirmative action is the way to go. 'Equal opportunity' on its own is just not enough. Corporations should be made to hire those with disabilities, and should be prevented from firing employees upon disablement. Affirmative action, she claims, may only be an incrementalist reform, but it has achieved results for other minorities.

Russell identifies the concept of equal opportunity, in terms of an anti-discrimination focus, within the competitive market system; that is, a system where there is supposedly no discrimination, but where the employer may choose the employee according to individual merit. Such an approach denies the structural relations that influence what is available to individuals, and even the very content of merit as a concept. Merit as a concept in most contexts carries a medical assumption of being able-bodied, thereby excluding all those labelled as living with a disability (see also President Obama's 'Disability Agenda' *White House—President,* 2009:1).

There is an argument that the third-way allows for a broad policy scope in terms of equality of opportunity. This is acknowledged by the differences in social policy between the political landscape of third-way in Germany and in the United Kingdom. In the United Kingdom, the practical pursuits of the third-way are aligned with left-leaning neoliberal and meritocratic theories of equal worth. On the other hand, Germany follows a more social democratic approach. The differences are linked to the UK's neoliberal political economic approach, which, it is argued, make neoliberal economics socially acceptable; while German social democratic politics recognise that the market will never create social equality (Russell, 2001a). Therefore, the German state has taken a more interventionist stance on equal opportunity. For example, the German government stipulates that employers with more than a certain number of employees must ensure that a given percentage of their employees are disabled, and this, we would say, is a form of affirmative action.

By contrast, the past Blair government in the UK took the view that equal opportunity is best served within society by meritocracy combined with equality of access. Blair argued that a meritocracy combined with equality of access provides for a society where there is equal worth, rewarding success for all regardless of their social background. This promoted the ideal that anyone can achieve success, unlike the earlier political stylings of aristocracy. According to Bacchi:

> Affirmative action is a controversial reform. Or at least, it is a reform that attracts great controversy. Its critics describe it as at odds with notions of equal opportunity and as undermining the procedure designed to appoint the best person for the job. Its supporters often, even usually, feel the need to qualify their support—to specify that *their* form of affirmative action does not undermine merit (Bacchi, 1996:1).

Even so, affirmative action may not be enough to allow people with disabilities to be granted employment. The costs associated with modifying equipment for people with disabilities are a hurdle for some companies. According to Russell (2001a:6), '[t]he disabled person's theoretical right to an accommodation is really no right at all; it is dependent upon the employer's calculus.' Russell notes that the bottom line in private business is to accumulate profits and pay the costs involved in making them. In the Australian context, this is noted by the *Disability Discrimination Act*'s hardship rule (Russell 1999b; 1999c; 2000a; 2001a).

Another policy approach to the employment of people with disabilities that should be discussed relates to the government fulfilling the role of employer of last resort.

A critical analysis of employment for people with a disability

> In order to bring more excluded persons into the workforce, it will be necessary to expand the work environment beyond the capitalist profit motive and ensure that federal and state governments act as the employers of last resort (Russell, 2000a:6–7).

The use of the government as employer of last resort is a cornerstone of full employment, acknowledging employment as a fundamental economic and human right. This basic idea is that the government employs anybody with an impairment, who is ready and willing to work at an appropriate wage, and who has been unable to find work through the private sector—the idea being that many government-controlled enterprises are capable of divorcing themselves from the profit-making cycle. Stretton (2005:83) describes the policy in this way: it is the 'consideration of [the] economy and humanity [which] should drive us to see that there is paid work for everyone who wants it.'

To give one example of this model in action, in 1983, as a person with a disability, I sought employment with the Australian federal government under a scheme designed specifically for people with disabilities. At the time, a government prescribed position, I believe, was the only major employer to whom a prospective employee with disabilities could apply without being stereotyped as non-functional, or as a liability likely to reduce an employer's profits. I gained employment by passing an intellectual testing process that was flexible within equal opportunity guidelines. The government has since continually reformed its program as employer of people with disabilities. Recently released Australian statistics, as reported by the Human Rights and Equal Opportunity Commission, attest to this:

> The number of people with disabilities employed by the Commonwealth government has declined significantly over the last ten years. In 2003–2004, people

with disabilities made up 3.8 per cent of ongoing Australian Public Service employees, down from 5.8 per cent ten years ago (Human Rights and Equal Opportunity Commission).

However, these approaches have faced challenges, not only from the private sector and from government, but also from within the disability rights movement. It is felt the acts of 'affirmative action' and 'government as employer of last resort' will promote discriminatory stereotypes and stigmas within the workforce, and that people with disabilities are only hired because it is so regulated. But these forms of discriminatory stereotype and stigma can be proscribed by legislation. In the long run this will promote the employment of people with disabilities as a societal norm.

There are many economic advantages to government being the employer of last resort. Forstater identifies its potential to supply full employment that will directly and indirectly help to assist other economic benefits, which include reducing economic fluctuations by promoting economic stability. One implication of the government as employer of last resort is that much of the budget currently spent on disability services pensions might be reduced or eliminated as there would be no need to totally fund such programs. As Forstater concludes:

> A primary reason for overlooking the advantages of public employment has been due to the tendency to evaluate public sector activity by the same criteria that private sector activity is evaluated. But public sector activity serves a different purpose than private sector activity and so should be evaluated according to different criteria. The public sector is not constrained by the same competitive pressures as the private sector, and therefore it has a greater degree of latitude in choosing what activities to engage in, what methods of production to utilize, and where to locate its activities (Forstater, 1998b:7).

Global neoliberal values combined with meritocracy has redefined the dominant political landscape, transforming the marketplace by focusing on individual merit and economic growth. However, many individual and market-based policies have been reviewed around the world, especially those countries affected by the global financial crisis. Economic growth has been assisted to a large degree by the technology boom, which has changed the way we communicate and work.

Neoliberalism, with its newly found focus on meritocracy, is said to have created new avenues to employment. Hence, the neoliberal features of technological and economic progress will allow for social inclusion in the workplace, especially for a determined few of those with disabilities (Stretton, 2002). The third-way advocates argue that it is defined by an era widely acknowledged to thrive on its new capacity for effective communication, opening up a range of possible employment opportunities for people with disabilities.

The third-way and neoliberalism have created the concept of a new form of political ethics, such as that of mutual obligation. A central principle of mutual obligation is concerned with a person's obligation to the State, which is created by the receipt of welfare benefits. This approach argues that the welfare recipient has an obligation to society to perform a duty for the benefits they receive. In short, welfare rights carry responsibilities (Pusey, 2002). However, it is argued that people should only be obliged to participate if offered work they can actually do, while noting that, currently, people with disabilities are not given support to find out if they can work, but rather for demonstrating that they can't.

Neoliberal policy reforms have evidently not shown that an economically efficient and pragmatic way of empowering welfare recipients is by ensuring that welfare rights carry responsibilities (Stretton, 2003). But, mutual obligation is not a sensible way to decide who is worthy, needy, or just greedy. Mutual obligation is paternalistic, and does nothing to assist those who need help in finding work.

A regime like this sends out a message detrimental to the social cohesion of all people. It asks 'how dare you claim benefits?', rather than 'can we help you to find work?' When it comes to people with disabilities, mutual obligation enforces a welfare system that many are unable to commit to, thereby creating further avenues of social exclusion.

The politics of mutual obligation compromises the ability of the government to fulfil its responsibility for the development of social cohesion among all of its citizens. This will affect society's capacity to work towards common goals, such as aspirations fundamental to the collective welfare responsibilities of the state. Therefore mutual obligation can affect society's social cohesiveness, which has a direct effect on the social inclusion of all, especially people with disabilities.

The neoliberal beliefs behind work and culture

Working within the community is an important part of social inclusion for many. People are defined by the type of work they do, which can enable mutual respect with others in society. This will also enable individuals to gain a certain level of income that will help develop a certain level of social inclusion. Being in paid work is the same as carrying a personal badge of honour, allowing greater personal self-esteem and social inclusion. However, most of the social democratic principles of the third-way are defused by the heavy reliance of neoliberal policies of the market and meritocracy.

Employment has changed in recent times, creating a shift in our understanding of paid employment. The workforce, in many cases, has been changed and challenged by the large-scale implementation of technologically inspired communication advancements. This has allowed some people, including those with disabilities, to operate advanced communication devices. This development of information and communication technologies has been argued, by western governments and their oppositions, to be inspired by market beliefs to drive the economy and an individual merit-based system.

Current political systems assume that manufacturing output will not decline but its workforce will, because most new jobs are created in the service sector of the economy. For example, information technology (IT) is now the single biggest sector in the US economy, constituting about 11 per cent of GDP (*Encyclopedia of the New Economy*, 2001, as cited in Gibilisco, 2011).

Where does this leave people with disabilities? This shift has changed the way we view the workplace. If you are a person with a physical disability in theory it is believed you potentially have a much greater chance of being employed than previously, because the new economy identifies itself more with brain power than with physical abilities, which in the past were the back bone of mass production (*Encyclopedia of the New Economy,* 2001, as cited in Gibilisco, 2011). But the third-way has only made the problem of employment for people with disabilities worse by its assumption that it is the change in technology that will create change in discriminatory practices and attitudes (Pusey, 2002). While the emergence of new technologies has the potential to improve the workplace experiences of people with disabilities, this will only occur if progressive social and political change also occurs.

It is argued that the third-way looks to efficiently and effectively improve the global spread of capital, which focuses on industrial production and competition. These are boosted by the development of new information and communication technologies, which draw on new kinds of labour that will put pressure on traditional styles of employment. Employers today and in the future will find themselves in a marketplace that must contend with intense competition on cost, quality, and flexibility of services. In such a context, the idea that the benefits of growth will trickle down to all, including people with disabilities, is severely limited.

Current trends towards individual merit in labour markets have brought about high levels of knowledge and adaptability in information and communication of skills. Such prospects may offer people with disabilities chances of employment that they may not have had in the past. Many authorities in western countries expect new social benefits to trickle down from economic growth driven by these technological advances. For instance, some theorists justify market-driven economic thought by believing that as the economy grows, the labour market grows as well, increasing the possibility that employers will employ additional staff to cope with increased business activity.

Economic growth also increases the capacity to fund social programs that will appraise the specialised and needed training of people with disabilities, so they may become an integral part of the workforce (Finn, 2002). An investment in human capital is the outcome of skills training in vocational subjects that promotes economic participation and social inclusion. Such an opportunity will stimulate the need for wider networks of support, which are a key to the disclosure of equal rights and opportunities for people with disabilities now and in the future.

The third-way identifies the need for national debates about social inclusion for all who can identify with the changes to work and training brought about by our global commitments. There is also the need to develop a strategy for helping people with disabilities and the non-disabled alike. This can happen through the implementation of policies that would enlighten and modernise the agendas of work and training for everyone.

Therefore, many economists will find it practical to acknowledge that as soon as people with disabilities and the non-disabled can be identified as those in the labour market capable of performing the job well, such job allocations will be able to serve as a self-regulating mechanism for wages, prices, and production. The economic demand analysis speaks of the need for workers trained in technological fields that will encourage more workers to seek such training, and eventually reducing wage inequalities.

Russell argues that such a neoclassical theory of competition holds that the labour market will eventually come to a point of equilibrium concerning pay rates and employment differentials. The initial inequality in pay rates can be explained as a result of the onset of supply and demand for information technology and a trained workforce, being one that is capable of creating differences in skills. This is acknowledged by the economic fact that those most trained in these new fields reap the benefits in pay from the transformation in the workplace, while those without such training fall behind.

Governments and their oppositions in the West have argued that the continuing development of advanced technology has been inspired by market beliefs that are driving the economy and an individual merit-based system, which is likely to advance our working and social inclusion. Technological progress is bringing a steady decrease in manufacturing work, and a fast increase of forms of work that are within the purview of our rising proportion of skilled and highly educated people, including many of those with physical disabilities. Some of these new jobs can be cheaply outsourced overseas. Most of them are in the service sector of Australia's economy. Protagonists argue that the current system of meritocracy is likely to distribute such skilled jobs and their rewards fairly enough to reduce, rather than increase, our inequalities.

Against this, Russell argues in the US context, which is relevant to most western countries:

> What happened instead is that government and the corporations abandoned American workers, including disabled workers, leaving them in the dust in search of

cheaper labour made possible by that very technology. Privatization of government jobs and IT outsourcing—sending jobs overseas—have become a popular means to lower the cost of labour committed to perform computer-related functions (Russell, 2004:1).

Russell identifies the current environment with new types of employment processes. Hence, in today's environment, it is cheap to outsource prospective jobs overseas to countries like India and Malaysia, and, soon, to China, where workers can be hired for about 10 per cent of the salary of a local employee, disabled or non-disabled (Russell, 2004).

Most of the employment that can be outsourced overseas is low-paid insecure work, such as data processing where the Internet is used to accommodate international transactions. The work that is being outsourced is employment being attended to, or that can be attended to, by many of our nation's people with disabilities (Russell, 2004).

Again, profit maximisation dominates over any ideas of social inclusion in the decision-making of corporations. Here, we see the political economics of neoliberalism at work, as employers seek to exploit labour on a global scale, searching for cheap labour wherever it is located and being supported by the neoliberal ideology of non-intervention in the market.

People with disabilities are, to a large degree, conceptualised as an exploitive product of the global, meritocratic and market-driven political economic system. This system is based on the ideal of profit making, not a dream that sees people interacting in the workplace with members of the so-called disabled body. In the long run, this will only permit the further exclusion of people with disabilities, promoting the economic conditions that are necessary to get rich by putting profit before people.

Works Consulted

ABS, (2012), Disability rate by age, Australian Social Trends, March Quarter 2012: *Disability and Work*, http://www.abs.gov.au/AUSSTATS/abs@.nsf/Lookup/4102.0Main+Features40March+Quarter+2012.

AIHW (2008) 'Trends in Employment', *Disability in Australia: trends in prevalence, education, employment and community living*, June, Bulletin 61, 22–28.

Sen, A (1999), *Development as Freedom*, Anchor Books, New York.

Bacchi, C (1990), *Same Difference. Feminism and Sexual Difference*, Allen and Unwin, Sydney.

Bacchi, C (1996), *The Politics of Affirmative Action*, Sage, London.

Human Rights and Equal Opportunity Commission (2005) 'National Inquiry into Employment and Disability', 1–8, http://www.hreoc.gov.au/disability_rights/employment_inquiry/papers/issues1.htm.

Clear, M (2000d) 'Appendix 3', *Promises Promises*, Clear, M (ed), Federation Press, Sydney, 175–176.

Cooper, J (2006), 'Inclusion our destiny?' *Education for tomorrow*, 88, http://www.educationfortomorrow.org.uk/2006/88inclusion.html.

Finn, D. (2002), Interview with Peter Gibilisco, unpublished.

Forstater, M (1998b) 'Flexible full employment: structural implications of discretionary public sector employment', *Journal of Economic Issues*, Volume 32, Number 2, 1–7, http://infotrac.galegroup.com.mate.lib.unimelb.edu.au/itw/infomark/42/305/60102805w4/purl=rc1_EAIM_0_A20970250&dyn=3!xrn_20_0_A20970250?sw_aep=unimelb.

Gibilisco, P. (2006b), 'Delivering employment to the disabled', *On Line Opinion*, November 22, 1–2, http://www.onlineopinion.com.au/view.asp?article=5140.

Gibilisco, P. (2011g), *Politics, Disability and Social Inclusion: People with different abilities in the 21st Century*, VDM Verlag, Saarbrücken.

Legal Aid, Victoria (2003) Using Disability Discrimination Law: a booklet for people who have a disability, Second Edition, 1–27, http://www.legalaid.vic.gov.au/upload/Disability_Disc rimination_2003.pdf.

Pusey, M (2002), Interview with Peter Gibilisco, unpublished.

Russell, M (1998c), *Beyond Ramps: Disability at the End of the Social Contract*, Common Courage Press, Monroe—Maine.

Russell, M (1999b), 'Government Example Setting Not Enough', Znet Daily Commentaries, 1–4, http://www.zmag.org/sustainers/content/1999-12/05russell.htm.

Russell, M (1999c), 'Productive Bodies and the Market', *Left Business Observer*, November, Number 92, 1–5, http://clem.mscd.edu/%7Eprincer/ant440b/article_prod uctive.htm.

Russell, M (2000a), 'The Political Economy of Disablement', *Dollars and Sense*, September, 1–7, http://www.disweb.org/marta/ped.html.

Russell, M (2001a), 'Disablement, Oppression, and the Political Economy', *Reinterpreting Disability Rights: Corporealities, Discourses of Disability*. University of Michigan Press, 1–35, http://www.martarussell.com/russell_umich_edit.html.

Russell, M (2003c), 'Backlash, the Political Economy and Structural Exclusion', in Linda Krieger, (ed.), *Backlash Against the Americans with Disabilities Act*, Number 21, 1–33, http://www.martarussell.com/papers/BJELL_EDIT. pdf.

Russell, M (2004), 'Capital Destroying Jobs ', Znet Daily
Commentaries, 1–3,
http://www.zmag.org/sustainers/content/2004-
03/04russell.cfm.

Russell, M (2000b), 'Why not capitalism', Z net: Daily
commentaries,
http://www.zmag.org/ZSustainers/ZDaily/2000-
05/20russell.htm.

Stretton, H (2002), Interview with Peter Gibilisco, unpublished.

Stretton, H (2003), Interview with Peter Gibilisco, unpublished.

Stretton, H (2005), *Australia Fair*, UNSW Press, Sydney.

The White House—President (2009) 'The Agenda—
Disabilities', 1–2,
http://www.whitehouse.gov/agenda/disabilities.

CHAPTER 6

Service Provision for People with
Severe Physical Disabilities

> That is law and that is dignified. A lift signifies that disabled are first class citizens with rights—not damaged goods—and able to board a bus without 'help' which is the old charity model of disablement. At least the IAC office did not patronize me and try to talk me into not going because it would be too difficult for me. I've had some do that. Their notion is that wheelchair users should not venture to go to Brazil or to Rome or to Genoa. Then when we are not there our views are silenced, we are not part of 'the people' the organizers speak about (Russell, 2003).

During the late 1960s, the Independent Living (IL) movement emerged in Berkeley, California, spearheaded by a disabled students' group known as 'The Rolling Quads'. It promoted the empowerment of people with disabilities and focused on dismantling the structural barriers imposed by the built environment, rather than focusing on the impairments of individuals. The first Centre for Independent Living, based on the social model of disablement, was founded in Berkeley and looked to broaden struggles for empowerment to include people with disabilities. Within a few years, hundreds of Independent Living Centres (ILCs) had begun across the United States, as well as a number of other countries including Britain, Canada, Australia and Brazil.

Despite the impressive work of such movements, Russell (1999a) argues that the increase in the population of people with disabilities of late has not been matched with increased funding in community care services in the United States and Australia alike (Gibilisco, 2003b; 2006c; 2007b; 2008b). Rather, there have been reductions in the size of the service provision side of the government and an increase in competitive orientated policy, which encouraged cuts to progressive social policies.

This chapter takes the example of service provision for people with physical disabilities from my home State of Victoria, as well as incorporating a discussion of support workers and their personal stories.

The Victorian State Disability Plan: reality or rhetoric?

The State Disability Plan 2002–2012

In its original formulation the State Disability Plan (2002) reflected the neoliberal ideology in its attempt to promote social inclusion for people with severe physical disabilities.

Key elements of this plan include:

> This State Disability Plan outlines a new approach to disability that is based on fundamental principles of human rights and social justice **(the way forward)**.The Principle of Dignity and Self-Determination **(choice)** is about respecting and valuing the knowledge, abilities and experiences that people with a disability possess, supporting them to make choices about their lives, and enabling each person to live the life they want to live **(guiding principles)**. This will ensure that real progress is made towards achieving the Government's vision over the next ten years **(next steps)** (Victorian State Disability Plan, 2002).

However, it is my experience that the State Disability Plan has had little positive effect upon the way support services are delivered for people with severe physical disabilities. Indeed, the practical implementation of the theoretical principles outlined in the State Disability Plan has in not a few cases caused confusion and may even have developed new forms of exclusion in these support services for those being served, their families and support workers. Considerable anxiety and frustration arises in everyday life when such support services are needed.

The disability plan 2013–2016

As a passionate disability advocate I would like to pose some critical questions. My concern is also about a practical and realisable theory in disability policy that takes into account the dynamic need for practical assistance with disability services. For example, bureaucracies can too easily generate fanciful justifications for innovations with their minimal budget. It seems that because of the many needs that have to be met with minimal resources a situation is created in which innovative but marginal projects are given priority.

The reality is that 45 per cent of those with a disability live in or near poverty, a rate that is more than 2½ times that of the general population. This places Australia as the worst performer, last out of the 27 OECD countries, a truly shocking statistic.

Currently, there seems to be the vibe that everything related to disability is improving. It may well be that inclusion seems to be improving for those with milder disabilities but this cannot be said for the rest of the disabled population in Australia. I have tried to indicate why it cannot be improving as long as an overall dilemma is created by claiming to increase social welfare provision when social services are being cut. In other words, this alleged improvement may only indicate that the problem in disability service provision is deepening rather than otherwise.

Disability Services—efficient, standardised, impersonal

The dominant ideas about economic policy owe much to the influence of the public choice school of thought, and to the general belief in neoclassical economics that competitive market forces, driven by individual self-interest, are capable of running the most efficient and fair economy. Self-interest is thus viewed as altruism (Stretton and Orchard, 1994).

Currently, the use of public policies that can directly affect social inclusiveness through the creation of social dilemmas, allows for the accumulation of individual selfishness in social policy. Further to this, Public Choice theory has taken on board some of the policy actions pertaining to social dilemmas. This believes that an even worse social dilemma can be created to cover up the first.

Bringing about an old adage; the best way to cover up a mess is by creating a bigger mess, close by.

Such unfortunate situations, can dramatically affect the burgeoning principle for equality of treatment and service within the disability sector. That is, current public policy is the main reason for such social dilemmas and further issues.

The interests that prompt our economic activities can include the joy gained from the work we do, the pride in doing it well, and in its value to others. Adam Smith knew much more than neoliberal economists do about the range of selfish, unselfish, shared and generous interests that motivate our economic activities. But neither he nor they give much attention to the possibility of society being inclusive for people with severe disabilities. For example, most people with severe disabilities need particular kinds of government intervention to help cope with the hardships and human problems created by disability, and exacerbated by various kinds of market failure.

American disability author and activist Marta Russell believes that neoclassical economists see the free market as an equaliser, in that when it expands the economy, all will share in its prosperity. Its rising inequality is indifferent; as a natural phase of the business cycle it is good for the market and society at large, promoting efficiency through standardisation (Russell, 1998a).

Victoria's *Disability Act 2006* was passed to further the Victorian government's commitment to its State Disability Plan. Is the *Disability Act 2006* just another social dilemma? After all, the initial set-up costs have taken vast amounts of money out of a shrinking budget.

Traditional social-democratic and progressive theories reject the notion that inequality is a necessary evil, and contend that sustained economic equality is desirable to maintain social stability and to promote justice and sustain political democracy. Traditional social democrats believe that the market is not self-regulating.

Government efforts to counterbalance the negative effects of supply and demand include spending to create more jobs, market intervention to equalise skills and increase job training, and legislation mandating equal access to jobs through civil rights and affirmative action.

Stretton outlines the traditional Social Democratic belief:

> Societies like ours needed to change some of their moral beliefs. Instead of replacing old morals by better ones, a lot of people were persuaded that societies didn't need moral beliefs any more. That is of course a moral belief with a vengeance and one which capitalists and intellectuals can exploit for fun and profit (Stretton, 1986:181).

Stretton believes that selfishness is a part of human nature, as is its opposite, unselfishness, which is directly related to much of what is good in society. Based on such thoughts is an ideological dilemma that troubles economic thinking today. Should the welfare sector become more efficient by developing a more market-like system that could supply and deliver individual social services to those in genuine need of them?

Stretton asks: how could individual preferences in practice produce workable public policies? The technical planning, budgeting and coordination that now strain the resources of elaborate public services would have to be designed instead by each voter as he or she registered his or her vote. Critics of existing public services want to privatise the social services that could in principle be paid for by their customers, as we have done with telephones, banks, electricity, public roads, rail and air transport, and some security services. But should this include hospital and medical services, and education for all, regardless of a person's capacity to pay?

As a particular example, there is a huge unmet need for disability services where politicians consistently use the old cliché of not having the money in the budget to solve the problems, while they find ways to waste the public's money by setting up new initiatives that are bound to fail. Disability services cannot responsibly be effectively systematised or standardised for the efficiency objectives of a purely competitive society. Efficiency of disability services is irrelevant in my case and for most people with disabilities who require services to live. Disability services can help to provide essentials of life to people who are severely physically disabled.

Are individualised services the answer to an ineffective disability system?

The downside of individualised social services

The dominant political agenda is ignorance of the belief that people cannot get ahead in life on their own, proclaiming the many positive actions that individualism can supply, all dressed in neoliberal political rhetoric. This is despite the fact that we are only human, and our behaviours and attitudes are formed by our environment. In most cases, despite the independence that an individual may have, or how they may struggle to acquire it, we are social creatures, and we have to work together in order to help each other. As humans, most of us are social animals and therefore need to be part of society, contrary to the individual rhetoric of the dominant neoliberal political agenda, shown, for example, in this statement by a figurehead of that agenda, Margaret Thatcher. Just like altruistic beliefs such as the fact that we need to look after ourselves and then, also to look after our neighbour instead there being a collective government experience.

The worldwide shift in support services for people with disabilities first took place in the 1980s, implementing a marketised style of reform in the disability sector. This involves the goal of delivering more efficient support services for people with disabilities, based on calculations that identify the most efficient use and, therefore, help pave the way for budget surpluses. In the 1990s, support services reforms to disability sectors around the world were driven by neoliberal and third-way political ideologies, which favoured the market and a minimalist approach to government that can be characterised as a strategy for the survival of the fittest.

This is highlighted by the political rhetoric of today, which can be identified by the individualised support services that are promised by Disability Services (an idiosyncratic name— Disability Services); that is, created by the neoliberal political environments, and further integrated into both major parties in Australia at federal, state, and local government levels.

The individualised rhetoric of neoliberal discourse is criticised by Hugh Stretton, who questions the ability of individually based social services to drive effective public policy. If it is believed that the policies are derived, one by one, from the citizens' voices, one issue after another, the social initiative will eventually stray from its original intentions (Stretton, 2007).

This prompts the question: is the promotion of individualised social services just another social dilemma? This is because it provides a paradox in its ability to practically provide services. This highlights some of the complexities that are involved when they adhere to political rhetoric and reform traditionally collective social policies, with their standardised, systematic and individualised approach to disability services. Disability services needs to promote the social inclusion of people with disabilities, rather than political rhetoric. Such political rhetoric can be identified in Victoria's State Disability Plan.

Being a person with severe physical disabilities in Victoria, Australia

Although, this took place 7.4 years ago, such political rhetoric has been a dominant factor in most of my life's actions.

In February 2007 I proclaimed an intense attack through *On Line Opinion*. I outlined once again my arguments in the hope that a logical person from within Victoria's Disability Services would listen to me. In spite of the everyday hurdles I face living with this chronically fatal progressive disease, I have lived most of my adult life independently in Dandenong, and I believe I have acted as a role model for many people with severe physical disabilities.

During this time I have always tried to play a good hand with the cards life has dealt me. However, the disease has significantly progressed since I first started living on my own in 1989; and from 2002 onwards the progression of my disease has increased rapidly. But now that I have my PhD I have harder yards to accomplish: that is to participate in the disability sector as a person with a PhD, with expertise in the area of the political economy of disablement. I also have much personal experience of public policy as it pertains to those with severe physical disabilities that could assist in shaping future directions of public policy. But my attempts to participate have been restrained by Disability Services, a division of the Department of Human Services (DHS).

In their wisdom, staff at Disability Services in the DHS have, yet again, refused me the necessary personal care hours I need to capitalise on my PhD within the disability sector, and also to help slow down my medical deterioration. This further throws into question the stated claims of the State Disability Plan to provide for human rights, dignity and self-determination, when people with severe disabilities are denied access to necessary personal care that would improve their quality of life (Gibilisco, 2006b; 2006c; 2007b).

The constant deterioration of my body is a direct effect of my disability, and has left me vulnerable, but not inadequate. For example, my vulnerability is due to a lack of assistance with my disability now that I am having a lot of trouble with life in general; and we should also add the life of an academic professional to this mix, a life to which I have unquestionably gained the right (Gibilisco, 2006c:2).

My problem arises in that I had applied for the provision of extra personal care (HomeFirst program) in 2002 and was informed by mail that I was on the urgent list in November 2002. To support my application, I produced, what was in my opinion, a *prima facie* account of my need for additional assistance, with the backing of references from people who are leaders in their respective fields (Gibilisco, 2003b:1; 2006b:45; 2006c:1).

In previous years, I was granted a sufficient number of hours of personal care to keep my head above water, even allowing for further deterioration in my condition. But at that time all I required to fulfil my initial needs was to maintain the ability to be an exceptional student (mostly working on the computer for eight hours a day). Since finishing my PhD, along with my physical deterioration, my personal care needs have dramatically changed. I made what I considered to be a reasonable request to Disability Services for additional personal care hours, comprising a support worker for personal care for 23 hours a week, for 26 weeks.

These hours are used to conduct life's bare necessities, such as, getting me in and out of bed, an enema procedure, my hygiene and meal preparation—I only eat twice a day, breakfast and dinner (refrigerated during the day and microwaved at night). I also sought a support worker to assist with fitness for one and a half hours a week, for 26 weeks. These hours are flexible but well short of what I require.

Much to my disappointment, Disability Services only approved the following: three hours a week of personal care, for community access (to attend disability conferences, forums and meetings, to follow up with my PhD studies and to offer myself as an outstanding scholar within the disability sector); two and a half hours of personal care for assistance with a hydrotherapy session once a month. The latter has great benefits: it just feels fantastic to stand of your own accord (even if it's only in a hydrotherapy pool). Equally, one hour of massage therapy a month is helpful because my muscles are tight from the disease and this is exacerbated with extra fitness training (Gibilisco, 2007b).

However, the support services are a long way from the stated goal of the State Disability Plan to 'focus on supporting people with a disability in flexible ways, based on their individual needs, so that each person can live the lifestyle they want to lead' (State Disability Plan, 2002).

Is there an obligation to people with disabilities? A key objective of the State Disability Plan is:

> To enable people with a disability to pursue their individual lifestyles, by encouraging others to respect,

promote and safeguard their rights and by strengthening the disability support system so that people's individual needs can be met (Department of Human Services:3).

Welfare, according to social democrats, should be distributed on a rights basis, as opposed to a needs basis. But, most third-way sympathisers bolster their marketised beliefs by arguing that traditional social democratic welfare policies are antiquated.

In an era where both parties have become worshipers of the market and are owned by investors and corporations, the matter has become bipartisan. Neo-liberal and Third-Way politics both replace redistributive goals with a market approach catering to business class needs and both adopt the supply-side theory that the economy is burdened by overly-generous welfare provisions which give too much security to workers. President Clinton explained his pro business agenda clearly when he said, 'The era of big government is over.' His motto became 'more empowerment, less entitlement' and his slogan 'from welfare to work' (Russell 2001b:3).

The importance of support workers for people with severe physical disabilities

A primary 'goal' of the State Disability Plan is to provide support, that is, to encourage people with disabilities to live their own lifestyle. This is referred to in the plan, as the pursuit of individual lifestyles. In the plan such a pursuit is linked to the worthy aspirations of the 'person-centred approach' (PCA). However, the goals of such an approach are shown to be somewhat idealistic when support services work with severe disablement, which covers a large portion of those needing support. In reality, the implementation of support for severe disablement is limited by political processes that require a standardised response.

People with severe disabilities want and are competent to perform the majority of human activities with the help of a skilled and empathetic support worker. The goals of Victoria's State Disability Plan are to ensure such needs are adequately met; at least that is what it implies.

These rhetorical goals are to provide a person who has a disability the required essentials that mean people with disabilities have choice. I can emphatically acknowledge that human assistance is the most flexible and capable method of support. For example, there are infinite amounts of human problems that arise, and by ensuring empathetic and pragmatic support, that is, by assisting in the implementation of the measures outlined in the SDP, pathways are opened to help people with severe disabilities reach their full potential whether in work, education or relationships. My support worker describes her role as follows:

> My name is Debbie Mackenzie and in the past I was the main support worker for Peter Gibilisco. In the past two and a half years my support role has increased, becoming more wide-ranging and flexible in the duties of personal care, through to challenges that have helped improve the quality of his life. The following explains how this has worked. I want to emphasise the importance of a person-centred approach in all practical aspects of support and personal care.

> When I first came into disability support I had no idea what to expect from the practical side of disability. There were many differences from what I was taught in theory, and since I come from the aged-care sector I

knew I would need to change my way of thinking in order to serve in the arena of disablement.

Initially, I did not understand how working within the disability sector could be so different, but I soon realised the differences were huge. They were huge in these ways: of course there is an age factor; but also there is a much more intense emotional factor. I could see there was so much more living to be done. For example, there needed to be more community inclusion and opening up of choices for living. This is known to have a positive effect, at least in Peter's case, and should greatly improve the lives of many directly affected by severe disability.

I attended Peter's PhD graduation at the University of Melbourne as his support worker. What a privilege that was, just to attend, and it was so inspiring to have the knowledge of the many obstacles Peter has overcome and while never forgetting the big picture! So, yes, this is the first image of what I could see of his 'dare to dream' approach to life!

Then gradual changes started to take place in Peter's life, such as the much required and fought for increase in the needed hours of human support services, through more flexible hours and a pragmatic person-centred approach. This was how my life started to evolve more around the study and the pragmatic diligence of disability work, and I loved it.

Peter was losing his ability to project his opinion at conferences and forums—his voice was weakening and his speech impaired and slurred. Therefore, Peter sought advice from those at ComTec, who helped him out significantly by installing programs on his laptop computer that could adequately project a suitable voice. The ability to communicate more freely at such events has considerably furthered Peter's self-esteem.

The boost Peter gained from technology also allowed him the ability to further his professional contribution in ways that a knowledgeable and empathetic support worker can readily assist. I learnt very quickly the required computer skills that would assist Peter's quality of life. However, no training can explain where the boundaries are: these I worked on myself to enable me to work in a professional, yet empathetic, manner.

I attended a study tour to Hawaii with Peter in 2008. I learnt so much from this experience and I have also attained many valuable attributes from the experience. It gave me the opportunity to work in Hawaii, and allowed me to gain the organisational skills to get him there and help him pursue his dreams. The trip took an entire year to plan, as there were so many obstacles to work through, but when I saw Peter's determination to get there and really enjoy it, this became a vehicle for change that drove me.

Attending conferences and forums with Peter empowered me; I wanted to learn so much more about the disability sector. I was a successful recipient of a Department of Human Services Scholarship to further my studies in disability work. I am a second-year student and with the assistance of Peter's mentoring skills I expect to complete this and further my career within the disability sector.

Related pitfalls in an American context—
some lessons to consider

In this section, I discuss the opinions of two highly intelligent people from the United States, each with severe disabilities, and look at the issue of how support workers are undervalued by many in society.

Dr Don Parsons is an outstanding independent scholar and author who was diagnosed with Friedreich's ataxia in 1971 and, despite this, graduated with a PhD in 1985, from the University of California, in Los Angeles (Parsons, 2007). Having endured such suffering, and with his knowledge of the progression of Friedreich's ataxia, Don is clearly entitled to the respect he has earned for his scholarly, candid hands-on views about the political economy of support workers. Don practically and intellectually believes that the ability of a person to effectively communicate and interact with their support worker is of the utmost importance. The disability system of support is focused on the wage relationship so a support worker should, in theory, provide the minimum of personal care and maintenance. All else is, he believes, due to the relationship that the disabled person can develop with his or her support worker (Parsons, 2007).

There are also certain constraints, usually in terms of time, that appear to be inherent in the system. For example, if a person in need of support wants to attend some conferences they may be unable to do so because he or she is unable to vary the established hours of work by the support worker to a sufficient degree (Parsons, 2007).

Professor Yvonne Singer also has important views concerning support workers. She has suffered with cerebral palsy since birth, leaving her severely physically disabled. Despite this she is currently an online professor at two universities in the United States (Singer, 2008). With piercing insight, she justifies the reasons for a shortage of support workers. She believes one of these is that the actions of a support worker are not given any value in society. Many in society do not value the disabled and, equally, do not value actions that help the disabled achieve (Singer, 2008). This is only further exacerbated by poor training methods, low salary and no benefits. Singer also commented on the poor work ethic of support workers within the disability industry, due in many ways to budgetary cuts and the flow-on effects of poor administration in the United States (Singer, 2008).

Australia benchmarks a sizeable portion of its disability policy to that of the United States, whether it pragmatically works or not. This prompts the question: are disability support workers as undervalued in Australia as their colleagues are in the United States?

Synergy and inclusiveness for people with disabilities

It is important to promote the dynamics of mutually beneficial partnerships between support workers and people with disabilities, people who rather than being merely disabled should be viewed as those with many different abilities.

This exploration considers some pragmatic examples that encourage the participation of these people in contributing to a more inclusive society. The underlying goal of mutually beneficial partnerships is to chart the further education of those directly and indirectly related to disability work. The aim is to identify the pathways of courteous, mutually beneficial and helpful relating and partnering. The pathway needs to be identified so that by travelling it together both parties (and all other parties) can truly share life together.

This partnering approach is currently being developed by the Learning Partnership Project, which consists of 10 diversely abled people, five people with disabilities or different abilities, and five support workers. The exchange of views developed a sense of comradeship, a truly empowering experience for such a diverse group. So the question arises: what benefits can such a partnership offer to the disability sector as a whole?

The potential benefits for developing such mutually beneficial partnerships are substantial. The flow-on will be to all those in society who are indirectly and directly related to disability. For example, there is an unlimited possibility for the transference of abilities, which will create a new potential for social inclusion of people with different abilities and support workers in a dynamic, merit-based society.

The synergistic outcomes that can flow from this form of flexible support can be demonstrated through my own (unpaid) work. Synergy is a term that is popular in most human resource management departments, and simply defined it means that the whole is greater than the sum of its parts, i.e.,

1+1=3: or in my case the synergistic partnership created by the role of a mutually beneficial partnership between a person with my specific abilities and my support worker, allows me to flourish in my role as a disability activist-cum-independent scholar.

For example, the synergy I gain through the intervention of flexible disability support provides me with the means to achieve many of my goals in life. This flexible personal care is needed to manage the complexities of infinitely varied human behaviours of those people with disabilities. It provides for a sustainable future in relation to my own desires and plans and also for many others with different abilities.

This is done through assistance that helps me attain my full human potential when and where my physical ability is lacking. For example, I suffer from a progressive illness that means a steady deterioration of my motor skills, which in turn leaves all my physical attributes severely disabled. However, I am still able to perform research and write articles at a phenomenal rate, beyond that of many paid workers in the disability sector. Basically, my performance is created through the synergy gained mainly through the work of my support worker.

This synergy explains the transformation that takes place in people with such different abilities and support workers, where the mutual benefits that occur will provide for a more proficient and humanly thoughtful disability sector, providing for a more inclusive society. Synergy becomes a fundamentally conscious event, which motivates, transforms and unifies all of life with a concerted and organised combination of such people of different abilities and support workers—this then, in my view, is the path to unify and enhance the disability sector.

Synergy for people with different abilities and support workers is about life chances and the creation of opportunities. Therefore, the essence of synergy is to value difference.

In *field's* (furthering inclusive learning and development) Learning Partnerships Project there was a need to look at the methods of training in support service personnel to be competent providers of disability services. There is a need to put more emphasis on pragmatic training, rather than following a systematic theoretical approach that has become far too technical and clinical and has forgotten to strive for excellence.

Hence, this approach assumes that attitudes are not to be recognised by a theoretically calculated skill level, since an attitude is a relationship that is the key to the skills acquired and applied.

As humans most people, including those we are concerned with who have such different abilities, lead lives that are too complex to be systematised. That is, one cannot expect people to have the same behavioural responses to different stimuli. Thus, support workers need to look pragmatically at the needs of people with such different abilities as they carry out their support.

However, this is not to discount or diminish contemporary training for support workers, since academic programs should be used to develop such positive pragmatic thought. Further to this is the case for policy. There is a website to promote mutually beneficial partnerships, ways of discouraging stereotypes and the respect of the diversity of disability, through methods that encourage a broad and collective approach to disability service provision. Mutually beneficial partnerships explore ways of developing policy. This was recognised in the underlying assumptions of Victoria's State

Disability Plan 2002–2012.

Thus, *field's* Learning Partnership Project offers further empirical evidence to support the goals of that plan. It aims to provide a strong and flexible agenda for change. It reaffirms the rights of people with a disability to live and participate in the community on an equal footing with other citizens of Victoria. This project has as its goal the further justification of much needed flexibility and inclusiveness to which the State Disability Plan appeals.

Field's Learning Partnerships Project's aim is, fundamentally, to explore and understand some deeper issues facing such differently and diversely gifted people. These issues are created by overloaded systems of support that are struggling to meet growing demand. Thus, the Learning Partnerships Project is synergistically implemented to improve the working relationship and lessen the demands upon the support workers.

Debbie Mackenzie, who has shown me and many others her human instincts concerning one of our calculated risks, states:

Most people involved in the network contributed with enthusiasm, but there were others who preferred to step back in fear that it may fail. I observed people not being able to comprehend how Dr Gibilisco, a person with such a severe physical disability, could undertake the trip; unfortunately, they let his disability get in the way of appreciating his capabilities. Also, there was incomprehension about me as the support worker. How would I be able to productively assist with the requirements of personal care while also assisting Dr Gibilisco with his research work and its complex demands (Mackenzie, 2008:1)?

This is a brief preview of a small and worthy contribution that is capable of helping us identify, while outlining some prevailing negative forms of sympathy (not empathy) towards people with severe disabilities or different abilities. While underlying some possibilities created through synergy and, hence, mutually beneficial partnerships, it is important to acknowledge the principle that creates order from disorder.

Labour shortage in the disability sector

There is an evident workforce shortage in the disability sector. The reasons for this, in theory, may be many, but if we are to look at it pragmatically we may soon come to see that this shortage has not been realistically faced. That pragmatic realism is what I wish to encourage with this brief exploration.

This shortage will very soon reach a crisis point; the problem needs to be addressed and cured, from a pragmatic standpoint, rather than merely remaining satisfied with policies that are captive to a remote theoretical overview. And if we can indeed overcome this person-power shortage the flow-on will be to all those in society who are indirectly and directly related to disability.

I have pondered for some time whether guidance to the disability workforce can be found from what I have referred to in some of my writings as the 'synergistic' outcomes that result from the interaction of people with disabilities and their support workers (Gibilisco, 2009).

These effective working relationships should be given the respect that is their due for their rightful contribution to models of leadership. Why are these highly successful working relationships so often below the radar when it comes to forming social welfare policies for the disabled? Could it be that these highly efficient working relationships are simply out of sight and out of mind? Is that why they seem to attract such a lowly status when it comes to the common ideas that are assumed to be relevant to making improvements in the disability workforce? Maybe we need to look again at the manuals that are written for workers and develop a distinctively new theory of management. Why not?

The synergistic approach I advocate might best be seen as a 'bottom-up' (inside out) approach to the management and organisation of the disability workforce. It will demonstrate public confidence in the abilities of the people who are served to exercise control over their own lives.

Let me try and explain this 'synergistic' model of workplace leadership in more detail. In order to make sure that this kind of model is flexible enough to allow change, even if complete change does not take place, the aim is to avoid an approach which sees the disabled person as a problem and instead reckon with such a person as a 'problem-solver', just like anyone else, and just like the support worker, as well. In this a 'synergistic' model develops a distinctive understanding of societal inclusion.

Please look to Amanda Gunawardena sub chapter on page 259.

In this context, synergy for the disability workforce is a way to provide the correct form of guidance for people with different abilities and support workers. To have a bottom-up approach is about life chances and the creation of opportunities. Therefore, by initiating a bottom-up approach we confront the support worker who sometimes sees him- or herself as a person languishing at the lowest grassroots level who then needs the disability sector for employment. We need to turn this around. In my view a synergistic approach to the disability sector is not just about better help for the disabled person—it is about raising the status of all involved, and ascribing due respect.

The disability sector should also look favourably at enhancing the talents of such people and encourage them with a future within the disability sector by establishing a workable bottom-up approach.

Among the many workers in the disability sector, there are

some who offer great support and some who offer inadequate support. As the population of support workers is currently small, it is evident that we need to increase the number of support workers in order to bring about a change and, thus, meet the crisis in the over-stretched workforce. Also, it is quite apparent that we need an inducement to boost and maintain worker morale.

The disability sector needs a root and branch overhaul in its workforce so that from its more practical grassroots level it will meet the sometimes overwhelming needs that cry out for attention.

If regulated properly, a bottom-up approach within the disability sector can help build ways to share and disseminate information and stories, so that people can gain inspiration and correction where they need to be put right. In this way community-based peer relationships can develop in both formal and informal ways. When people are truly supporting each other and are aware that they indeed need each other's support then this leads to greater independence and perhaps even a trimming of the hard edges of the workload. Those working in the sector must suffer stress and yet a 'synergistic' approach that understands how the person served can also be stressed by the support worker's stress, may well be inclined to develop a more realistic approach for all involved.

Of course, we need to increase the practicality of the State Disability Plan so that people with disabilities are more fully able to publicly acknowledge the vital assistance they receive from support workers. For example, the implementation of disability support worker awards will also help DHS to get a handle on the quality of work and the workers, and learn to assess the skills that are of greatest use in the sector by taking a lead from the people who know—the people who are served and who can see with their own eyes the great support that is rendered.

This kind of morale-boosting reward system would have a positive impact on the disability workforce, thus boosting the work carried out by the support workers. The sector needs to find ways to support its best workers, and to encourage those who don't know how to offer what is truly needed.

However, each individual support worker should be judged on his or her merits. But this innovation may have teething problems, though this is to be expected. It may be true that workers also need further education—for example, in skills, legal aspects and other matters. Yet in many cases support workers have demonstrated their capacity of compassionate and wise support before they go on courses and they have thereby shown that they are already good workers within Disability Services. The key idea for this is: don't forget to ask the person who knows—the one who is on the receiving end of the support that is offered!

A reform Disability Services needs to push

Direct payments cuts (DHS, 2012), the financial costs and messy paperwork associated with disability supports, have changed the financial middleman and put some control over how the state government's Disability Services' money is spent. It places it directly into the hands of the disability support users.

Direct employment (DHS, 2012) takes direct payments further, by allowing the person with disabilities, family or a trustee to be an employer and administrator of his or her own support workers (disability supports).

For the 2012 state-wide implementation, direct employers are not allowed to set up as a business due to changes in the rules of the Australian Taxation Office. This is because 'individual support' funding will be treated as income for the business and attract tax, which will reduce the amount of funding available to purchase supports. People who have an individual support package (ISP) and are using direct payments can apply for 'direct employment' by contacting their local departmental office directly, or they can apply for direct employment at the next planned review of their individual support package. People who have an individual support package administered through the financial intermediary or a disability service provider can apply for direct employment but this will require a review of their individual support package and a change of funding administration to direct payments. People who have been allocated an individual support package for the first time, and who are confident they can fulfil the obligations relating to direct employment, can nominate to use direct payments and apply for direct employment in their first plan. Upon approval of the application, the signing of Direct Payments Agreement and Direct Employment Agreement, and the completion of an insurance application will be required. Therefore, a large amount of money is put into the training of disability professionals. But there is little credit given to the ability of people with disabilities, who often act in management roles, for the day-to-day management of their home-based support workers, or the management of disability professionals.

Direct employment gives people with a disability a degree of flexibility regarding the choice of support workers, negotiation of salary and hours, and work that needs to be undertaken. It also means that the hours of duty and pay rates become more flexible, too, which is more attractive to support workers. As a direct employer, the person with a disability will need to be familiar with a range of things, such as WorkCover and taxation laws. This can be complicated and may mean that they need to ensure they comply with legal, financial and human resource obligations, as well as maintaining employees' records. This may be related to type of work performed, hours of work, superannuation and tax details. The Australian Taxation Office's online tax withheld calculator can assist direct employers in meeting their taxation requirements. Employers must understand their insurance requirements and must continue to hold insurance through the Victorian Managed Insurance Authority (VMIA).

They must also have a WorkCover policy that insures their workers in the event that they are injured in the workplace. The forms that are needed to get started can be ordered or downloaded from the Australian Taxation Office's website.

Direct employment practices the belief that the people being supported are, more often than not, the best teachers regarding the support they need and how it can be delivered.

In short, whether through a financial intermediary or direct payments, you are locked into paying your service provider close to or the full amount of the hourly rate of $39.80 per hour, provided by Disability Services. Yet, Disability Service providers only pay support workers a meagre portion—about $20 per hour.

Therefore, the amount of around $19.80 per hour is quite substantial and should be used for what it was intended—rather than being used to pay a hierarchy of administrative wages for the service providers.

Direct employment, is to ensure that financial control of the supports being used is in the hands of people with disabilities, their family or their trustee. They will have far less overhead costs and can look at increasing workplace morale by increasing wages and/or increasing the work hours available.

And so, Disability Services will be asking people with disabilities, family or trustees, to take on these roles, sharing their know-how and experience when it comes to disability supports—something that usually takes a disability professional many years to achieve through training.

Often, the need for disability support is stretched beyond the means offered by government and NGOs. Individuals and groups are left needing disability support at times when the service fails to keep up with growing need. Direct employment develops the empowerment of people with disabilities by giving them more control over their disability supports. Also, this will give them the ability to build up responses to problems faced by many individuals with disabilities, as well as their families, friends and community.

Direct employment can build ways to gain information about how people can use community-based peer relationships, such as the necessary communication requirements and other methods that can be used to support each other. This can lead to a greater independence and a trimming of the workload and stress on those with growing needs for disability supports.

The successful development of peer support will allow for necessary forms of queries to be handled by peers who have succeeded in the same or similar circumstances.

Direct employment gives confidence and control to people with disabilities over their own lives, which is based on logic and social coherence. In order to make sure that this kind of model is flexible enough to allow change, even if complete change does not take place, the aim is to build flexibility into disability supports to bring the disabled closer to societal inclusion.

The empowerment of people with disabilities is the goal that helps the drive for success in providing a lasting improvement into the way disability supports are given: it changes the way in which trust is given for the provision of this. Direct employment will hopefully cut the costs and 'mess' in the provision of disability supports and build up solutions for the problems within.

The risks to direct employment

One of the risks to direct employment concerns the employment of support workers.

The uncertainty related to payments to support workers is a current concern. Prospective direct employers need to consult the Direct Employment Resource Guide, which advises people to think about what Award should apply to the work to be performed. The Resource Guide advises that in most situations the Social, Community, Home Care and Disability Services Industry Award 2010 rate will apply, but it is recommended that employers seek advice from Fair Work Australia. It is important that while Awards outline the minimum rate of pay, employers can always offer above that if they think it is necessary to attract and retain the right people. This must be managed from within the individual support package allocation. From an employer's perspective, paying employees at a casual rate brings about convenience to the direct employer in terms of arranging payments.

Direct employers are required to be familiar with a range of legal responsibilities, such as WorkCover and taxation laws. This can be quite complicated and may mean that you'll have to register with the Australian Taxation Office (ATO) for things like paying withholding tax. With pay withholding the direct employer is responsible for calculating how much tax to withhold from their employees pay, and is then responsible for paying this amount to the ATO. With direct employment, there is no legal requirement to do police checks, but direct employers may choose to conduct them.

There are also the concerns from the employee's perspective about the competence of disabled direct employers to perform legal responsibilities at the optimum level. The department does not know of, or suggest any, Occupational Health and Safety training or indeed any other training suitable for direct employers. Individual direct employers may decide that they would like this and so will need to make their own enquiries. However, there is a one-off grant of $500 for new direct employers that can be used for training to help a person establish themselves as a direct employer. Beyond that, any training would be paid for by direct employers out of their ISP. The $500 grant has only been a new incentive for direct employers, which was not available during the pilot program.

The $500 grant is not restricted to being used for training. People have the discretion to use it for anything that would benefit them in setting up their direct employment. For example, some have used it for purchasing bookkeeping software, and so on. The relationship between employer and employee (known as the employee relationship) is two-way. While the employer has many responsibilities, including the legal ones, employees also have responsibilities. This includes being confident prior to signing an employment agreement and/or commencing work that they will be able to work with the employer. Of course, despite their best efforts of finding out, situations may arise where the employee has concerns about how the employer is performing their responsibilities or treating them. It is up to the employee to work out a resolution. Where they go will depend on the issue. For example, if it is about pay and conditions they may talk to the Fair Work Ombudsman.

Help available to direct employers

Web2Care is a technological support platform launched in May 2007 by people promoting self-directed care as a future direction for individuals with complex care needs. The project is supported by DHS in Victoria. The development team is made up of care recipients and family members of persons with disabilities. Great difficulties with the current care delivery system and the common needs were identified by this development team. The care delivery process is improved and a comprehensive, end-user–focused Internet-based care management support system is developed through the use of latest Internet technology (Web2Care, 2012).

The Good Life Cooperative is an initiative of the National Steering Group on Self-Directed Services and Personal Budgets. It is a tool for making self-direction work on a large scale in disability. Their aim is to self-direct support to Australians with a disability who hold an ISP without the need for a service provider to deliver services to them. The Cooperative has four categories of members who collaborate to pursue their goals, such as individuals and families in receipt of care and support packages, coaching and coordination of organisations who support individual package holders, support workers who are committed to working in a personalised way; and technical intermediaries who are committed to self-direction. The program uses the Web2Care technology platform for self-direction (Good Life Cooperative, 2013).

Direct employment can build ways to gain information about how people can use community-based peer relationships, such as the necessary communication requirements and other methods that can be used to support each other. This can lead to a greater independence and a trimming of the workload and stress on those with growing needs for disability supports. The successful development of peer support allows for necessary forms of queries to be handled by peers who have succeeded in the same or similar circumstances.

Case studies

Peter Sember, a direct employer

Peter Sember is a direct employer who has a physical disability related to spinal muscular atrophy. Some of his thoughts on direct employment are:

'I don't need supports to be there all the time, but thanks to direct employment, they are there when I need them to be there,' says Peter Sember.

When Peter Sember's elderly parents were unable to continue providing him with 24-hour support, he needed a system of supports that could work around his full-time job and busy social life.

'Until four years ago, all my support was provided by members of my family so I didn't need any external supports,' says Peter. 'When my mother passed away, my father, who is 88 years old, was unable to provide me with the support I needed, so I needed to create a system that would be responsive to my needs. Working full time means I need personal support at 5.00 am to get ready for work. Before I started direct employment, the earliest time I could get a worker was 6.30 am or 7.00 am. It just didn't work.'

'I have all sorts of interests—friends, dinners and movies. With direct employment I can do a three-worker split shift, which allows me to do these things. On Tuesday nights, for example, I need to be driven to the city to have dinner with friends and then that worker goes to another job. I'll then need someone to help get me home, which is the second worker, and then a third worker attends and transfers me to bed. I don't need the workers all the time, but they are there when I need them to be.'

While Peter says direct employment suits his lifestyle, he warns that a certain level of skill and coordination is required. 'Some of the basic things that need to be in place are worker insurance cover, public liability insurance and pay-roll,' says Peter. 'These were the biggest hurdles.'

'The skills I've acquired in my full-time job, such as computer skills and problem solving, are all used in direct employment. You have to be organised. It's almost like running a small business.' (Department of Human Services (a), 2012)

Amanda Gunawardena, an academic support worker

'My name is Amanda Gunawardena and I am an academic support worker at the University of Melbourne. I assist direct employers like Peter with computer-based administrative tasks.

'I am keen and supportive of direct employment as it offers me flexibility with the type of work and working hours. I can adjust my work schedule according to the availability of other workers and also my personal commitments. This means that I can be there for work, and for my family when they need me. I also feel like it gives me a sense of dignity in my role seeing that I am helping the empowerment of people with disabilities.

'As I help Peter perform administrative duties that are related to direct employment, such as taxation payments, it has been a learning experience for me. I am now aware of many things that I didn't [sic] before, such as legal responsibilities of an employer. Peter's knowledge and my abilities combined together generally produces fast, efficient and improved results as can be noted throughout this book. Peter has a lot of intelligence and expertise in the field of his study, but his abilities to put his thoughts to words is restricted by his slow typing speed, poor speech and eyesight. However, when I am there to assist him, this means that he can get his thoughts on paper at 50 words per minute.'

Ajay Joseph and Cunxia Li, support workers

These are some thoughts from Cunxia Li and Ajay Joseph, two support workers for Peter Gibilisco:

'We are supportive of direct employment, and think it has many benefits. We think direct employment is the best option for the people with disabilities. Funding from DHS is spent mostly for administration when considering living in support accommodation or using service providers for one-on-one support. But, by using direct employment, people with disabilities can choose their own support staff they like, and use most of the funding for their support work if they choose to. You can help the people with disabilities lead their own lives and help them make decisions for themselves. Direct employment meets individual needs and suits individual lifestyles, which makes it very suitable for people with disabilities. We think "person centred" just means "direct employment".

'But we do have concerns as well. We'll be [sic] concerned on how Occupational Health and Safety procedures and risk assessments are done in direct employment and also on how they get updates on Occupational Health and Safety policies. The awareness of employers of all the legal responsibilities and also if they are able to successfully complete them is one of my major issues. We're interested to find out how the employers are trained into assisting those—becoming confident employers. Job security and also awards and wages [are] something to think about in this context.

'Direct employment's flexible approach to disability support may help sway and bring about mutually beneficial partnerships that are created by the working relationship between direct support workers and people with disabilities. This is noted by the term "synergy theory", which is said to help people with disabilities to become people with different abilities.'

Works Consulted

Cooper, J (2006). Inclusion our destiny? Education for tomorrow, 88, http://www.educationfortomorrow.org.uk/2006/88inclusion.html.

Department of Human Services (a). (2012), Direct Employment Resource Guide. Accessed 10th August 2013 from http://www.dhs.vic.gov.au/about-the-department/documents-and-resources/policies,-guidelines-and-legislation/direct-employment-resource-guide.

Department of Human Services (2012a), 'Direct Payments', Department of Human Services website, http://www.dhs.vic.gov.au/for-service-providers/disability/self-directed-support/direct-payments.

Department of Human Services (2012b), 'Evaluation of the Direct Employment Project: Disability Services', Department of Human Services, http://www.dhs.vic.gov.au/about-the-department/documents-and-resources/reports-publications/evaluation-of-direct-employment-project.

Gibilisco, P. (2013), Interviews with Amanda Gunawardena, Ajay Joseph and Cunxia Li, unpublished.

Gibilisco, P. (2000), 'The Cost Disease caused by Public Choice Theory'. Hugh Stretton and the social sciences (Masters Thesis) pp. 75–82.

Gibilisco, P. (2003c), 'A Study in Success', *Campus Review*, Volume 13, Number 25, July 2nd–8th, 9.

Gibilisco, P. (2006c), 'Social inclusion for the disabled is a mirage', *On Line Opinion*, August 8, 1–2, http://www.onlineopinion.com.au/view.asp?article=4746.

Gibilisco, P. (2006d), 'The State Disability Plan—Rhetoric and Reality', *Just Policy*, March Edition 39, 44–49.

Gibilisco, P. (2007b), 'Disability Services—efficient, standardised, impersonal', *On Line Opinion*, August 16, 1–2, http://www.onlineopinion.com.au/view.asp?article=13142.

Gibilisco, P. (2007c), 'The downside of individualised social services', *On Line Opinion*, October 30, 1–2, http://www.onlineopinion.com.au/view.asp?article=6572.

Gibilisco, P. (2007d), 'Wasting expertise and wasting lives', *On Line Opinion*, February 28, 1–2, http://www.onlineopinion.com.au/view.asp?article=5545.

Gibilisco, P. (2009a), 'Achieving a synergy for the disabled', *On Line Opinion*, 19 May, 1–2, http://www.onlineopinion.com.au/view.asp?article=8873.

Gibilisco, P. (2011b), 'A reform Disability Services needs to push', *On Line Opinion*, 20 December, 1–2, http://www.onlineopinion.com.au/view.asp?article=13 017.

Gibilisco, P. (2011e), 'Labour shortage in disability sector', *On Line Opinion*, 17 November, 1–2, http://www.onlineopinion.com.au/view.asp?article=12 892.

Gibilisco, P. (2012), 'The State Disability Plan: reality or rhetoric?', *On Line Opinion*, January 19, 1–2, http://www.onlineopinion.com.au/view.asp?article=13 142&page=2.

Gibilisco, P. and Mackenzie, D. (2009), 'Mutually beneficial direct support partnerships—Key to satisfaction for a more skilled and longer lasting workforce', NDS Conference, May 4, Hotel Grand Chancellor: Hobart.

Gibilisco, P. (2013d), 'Direct employment: by and for people with disabilities', *On Line Opinion,* August 28, 1-three[fix], http://www.onlineopinion.com.au/view.asp?article=15 400

Gippsland Carers Association (2011), "State Disability Plan 2013–2016", Gippsland Carers Association website, November 19, 1, http://www.gippslandcarers.org/state-disability-plan-2013-2016.

Good Life Cooperative. (2013). Co-Op Home. Accessed 8th August 2013 from, http://www.goodlifecoop.org/.

Mackenzie, D. (2008), 'Overseas Research Trip', *Not Just Work*, November 18, 1–2, http://notjustwork.info/archives/overseas-research-trip/.

Parsons, D. (2008), Interview with Peter Gibilisco, unpublished.

PWC (2012), 'Disability in Australia: What needs to change
    if the NDIS is to make a meaningful difference?',
    PWC website, July 12, 1,
    http://www.pwc.com.au/industry/government/publicati
    ons/disability-in-australia.htm.

Russell, M. (1998c), 'Persistent Inequalities', DisWeb:
    socio/economic aspects of disablement pp. 1–5,
    Downloaded to Word,
    http://disweb.org/marta/pov.html.

Russell, M. (1999), 'George W. Bush Y2000?', Znet Daily
    commentaries;
    http://www.zmag.org/ZSustainers/ZDaily/1999-
    10/1russell.htm.

Russell, M (2001b) 'What's Wrong with "Charitable
    Choice"? A Plenty', *Znet Daily Commentaries*, 1-5,
    http://www.zmag.org/sustainers/content/2001-
    03/28russell.htm

Russell, M. (2003). 'The People' Speak Out. *The freedom and justice crier.* 11. Accessed 7 February 2014, http://www.neym.org/PrejudiceAndPoverty/Issue11.summer2003.pdf.

Singer, Y. (2008), Interview with Peter Gibilisco, unpublished.

Stretton, H. (1986), 'Foreword', in Wilenski, P. Public Power and Public Administration, Hale and Iremonger, Sydney, 7–9.

Stretton, H. (1997), Interview with Peter Gibilisco, unpublished.

Stretton, H. (2007), Interview with Peter Gibilisco, unpublished.

Stretton, H. and Orchard, L. (1994), Public Goods, Public Enterprise, Public Choice: *Theoretical Foundations of the Contemporary Attack on Government*, St Martins Press, New York.

Victorian Department of Human Services (2002), Disability Services Division. Victorian State Disability Plan 2002–2012 Disability Services Division, Dept. of Human Services, Melbourne.

Web2Care (2013). Web2Care: Technology Support for Self Directed Care Programs. Accessed 9th August 2013 from http://www.web2care.net/.

CHAPTER 7

Pushing for justice: the author interviewed by Bruce Wearne

Foreword (by Bruce Wearne)

In the pages that follow, Peter tells his own story while issuing a call for greater awareness of the task of ensuring that safe and just structures of care prevail for those whose abilities to contribute are severely constrained by bodily malfunction, disease or injury.

I have known Peter for over 20 years, since he first knocked on my door at the Frankston Campus of Monash University. He asked to be included in an 'Introduction to Sociology' summer semester course I was teaching. One thing led to another and, as he tells it, this enthusiastic student eventually concentrated on sociology and even developed the outrageous long-term aim of bringing the disciplines of sociology and economics together in some kind of creative symbiosis. These days he would say that sociology and economics need to overcome a loss of 'synergy'. But that was the start of our friendship. First it was as lecturer and student; then I became supervisor when he was an MA dissertation writer. Since then, Peter has gone on to gain a PhD, and a reputation among prominent economists for his brazen unwillingness to allow his condition to prevent his mobile mind from pushing ahead and knocking on doors around the country. More recently, I have acted as his proofreader and as colleagues we are joined as members of this Australian political community in doing what we can to promote public justice. So, that is why I am as qualified as anyone to probe Peter about his motives and I have done so in the following interview.

In closing this foreword, let me simply draw the attention of readers to Peter's attitude to social and political life. Not everyone can publish material that openly draws attention to his or her own bodily constraints. Of course, these are deeply personal issues. But Peter has learnt to write about his own responses to his progressive condition without worrying too much about the image he presents of his situation on the page, or, computer screen. There is something truly inspiring here and I would invite readers to think deeply about this problematic as they consider Peter's persistent push for justice for the severely disabled. The chapters that he has written for this book draw upon his own experiences and he contributes knowing deep down that much more is at stake than merely ensuring his own comfort.

Well done, Peter. Keep on pushing!

Bruce C Wearne

Point Lonsdale

Tuesday, November 20, 2012

Social space with economic room to move

Introduction

I am an advocate for the seriously disabled. Now for those who know me that may not come as much of a surprise. They know the condition that has affected me like a pain in the backside for decades. But as my condition has progressed so has my eagerness to act as advocate. First, a word of explanation before we begin.

This interview was initially sparked by my dissatisfaction with my own situation. Being dissatisfied with my situation is not new to me. I have had to give voice to my dissatisfaction ever since contracting Friedrich's ataxia at age 14. Nowadays, I find it even more difficult to communicate and that makes the dissatisfaction grow. My typing used to be two words a minute. That's no longer possible. I have asked my friend Bruce Wearne to assist me. Knowing my situation, and my concerns, he suggested this interview. By tossing these issues around we can explore the social context in depth and identify some aspects of caring for the disabled that are too easily overlooked. Then with his help in editing what I have said already in what I have published, I can put forward my views in a way that will not only emphasise the need of severely disabled people like myself for 'space with room to move', but can also take the role of 'disability consultant' to render advice to those who have to confront and resolve complex managerial issues that cannot be avoided when care is given. I know about these issues. I have studied them, first when I started a business studies course at Dandenong TAFE back in 1985. I did this course having 'come down to earth' and realised that creating a future for myself meant that I had to stop living in a fantasy world. You can read more about my ongoing efforts to come to terms with the 'pain in my backside.'

I don't want sympathy. I like to think that one of my skills, which I share with many others, is dodging the **sympathy** people instinctively have and instead I seek to promote **empathy** among members of our society. The creation of a just society requires the recognition of all members of society and their many and varied relationships, including direct and indirect involvement with political processes.

So here goes. Bruce, what's the first question?

Bruce: Peter, let's begin by talking about space and movement. These are basic aspects of everyone's life. But since you were 14 your body has suffered a condition that changes your view and constricts your experience of space and movement. Can you tell us a little about how this has happened?

Peter: I have had to struggle with Friedreich's ataxia since I was a teenager. I was 14 when this was diagnosed. It is a progressive disease, causing impairment to the nerves and, so, a failure of timely muscle reactions throughout my body. The messages sent from the brain via neurotransmitters are slower and weaker than they should be.

Bruce: And so, muscular growth is hampered, giving rise to various bodily problems.

Peter: Problems but let's not have any fantasy about this— these are severe deformities that I've had to learn to live with. It's a condition that increases my limitations as I live longer. For example, I have had to deal with severe scoliosis and cardiomyopathy. By 23, I was reliant upon a wheelchair, but now I'm simply too uncoordinated to make use of an electric one.

Bruce: So that means you need help in just moving: activity that people usually take for granted.

Peter: That's right. But remember what I said about 'empathy' instead of 'sympathy'. See sub chapter 'Empathy not Sympathy helps Inclusiveness' in Chapter 5.

Bruce: Let's come back to everyday movement issues after we explore this important distinction you make. Can you give me an example of where 'sympathy' is like a kick in the guts?

Peter: Yes. I completed my PhD six years ago, and I tried to gain employment within the not-for-profit disability sector. I applied for some positions that I was very well-qualified to fill. Take for example one position where the pay was very minimal for 20 hours per week at $20 per hour. Even in the sector the response was very unsatisfying.

Bruce: Are you just complaining that you didn't get the job?

Peter: Well yes and no. You confront a mindset. There's always lots of sympathy. But to employ someone with my qualifications, even in the disability sector, requires a structure that is empathetic. Budgeting needs to think about employment that would require a Personal Assistant even for a basic position. So it is structural, but it is very personal when you have to deal with being told your application is not successful.

Bruce: And then you are saying that sympathetic structures are such that your condition gives selection committees an opportunity to trim the list.

Peter: Exactly. Sometime after another failed application I learnt the following: 'Having interviewed Peter for a temporary job, his disabilities made it difficult to employ him despite his insights and contacts' (Media Player, 2008). That was a response to one of my *On Line Opinion* articles regarding employment in the disability sector.

Bruce: So you're sure that the person who wrote that was full of 'sympathy'. But making you a hero for not getting the job doesn't get you very far does it?

Peter: Exactly. It has been 20 years' hard work, in that case for not much at all: just another humiliating comment which lacks empathy.

Bruce: You mean that by putting it online in response to what you wrote it actually does the opposite of what the person intended to say?

Peter: I guess so.

Bruce: OK. Let's take this distinction between *sympathy* and *empathy* that is so basic to your push for justice.

Peter: Fine. Fire away.

Bruce: Well let's discuss getting out of bed, or getting into bed for that matter. As your condition has progressed, this means that you have needed more and more assistance. We won't go into all the messy details although I get it can easily get messy for you.

Peter: Sure. Yes let's keep to say the sociological and economic aspects of what's needed.

Bruce: How do you mean, Peter. Is getting out of bed and going to the toilet a matter of sociological and economic significance?

Peter: Of course. You taught me that. What happens to people like me with staff shortages? Or say there's some staff problem. Do I have to wait for six hours between shifts to urinate? Or think of what might happen in terms of rashes between my legs if somehow things get out of hand? If my skin gets infected I am in a lot of trouble.

Bruce: So you're saying that if places like where you are living now are registered as institutions that care for people like yourself, they have to be able to do so.

Peter: That's it. Because my condition has progressed I have had to learn patience and truly I am a pretty patient person. I do try to stay positive. I can't exactly throw a tantrum. But I have lived with this for a fairly long time already, for over 36 years, seven days a week in fact.

Bruce: Now you're a PhD and you've obviously been so expertly trained in sociology (Ho! Ho!) to closely observe the things that go on around you. I've also been trained in this way! And what you say about the need for a structural dimension to empathy is very important, I think. But in recent months I've observed that your emails have had an edge to them that I hadn't ever noticed before. I mean one of the things I have always noticed about you is your happy-go-lucky demeanour. Now as your condition progresses I guess it's natural to get frustrated. But, tell us a bit about these recent frustrations. I think the people who are reading this might benefit if you do so. It might stimulate a better understanding of the empathy that is needed.

Peter: Here's not the place to go into all the details of rights and wrongs. I'll give a few examples of problems I have noticed that irritate me.

Bruce: Go ahead.

Peter: Take for instance my academic support worker, Amanda. She does a lot of work for me. But such support is not mechanical like a cog that can be replaced. She's a person. My typing speed is a real pain in the ass. I cannot do what I want to do; I have to rely very much on Amanda to do the typing. Now this has also shown me the importance and potential of 'synergy' developing between people. Now you can say that all she does is my typing, but if she was to be replaced I would lose that relationship, that's synergy.

Think about my support workers. There are constant changes in my support workers. Why is this? It seems to me that 'He or she is only a support worker!' is a stereotype just as bad as 'Oh he or she is disabled!' Such shallow thinking actually destroys the potential of developing synergy. It also means that empathy won't get a look in. To put this in economic terms: the 'personal aspects' are reduced to 'disutilities' and therefore can be disposed of.

Bruce: So, by continuing to write you are actually trying to show 'empathy' for management and those who work with you, even if, as you repeatedly have pointed out in your articles that they have to work under the very dehumanising restrictions imposed by neoliberalism!

Peter: I'm just as selfish and self-oriented as the next person. I just really try hard not to take any notice of actions that are based on stereotypes.

Bruce: But you have. You are. You've been really irritated.

Peter: I guess so. But as my disability gets worse, I find it harder to avoid the stereotypes. I am very much aware of how negative, and emotionally and socially destructive they can be. So, I will still always be trying my hardest to combat stereotypes. And as I said, I am also aiming to improve social awareness through my writing.

Bruce: So, Peter, here you are in a 24/7 care facility—with all of its strengths and weaknesses—and some of the problems you've been facing, how do you, as a resident, think you are being treated here as a highly qualified 'disability consultant' from Melbourne University?

Peter: Good question. Let me refer to issues of safety for example. Some of these are treated in my *OLO* article about the 'dignity of risk'. But there are other sides to this.

Bruce: You've mentioned to me the contentious issue of your sling. You've used your former sling for a long time.

Peter: Yes, let's take my sling as an example. I used that old sling when I was being lifted in and out of bed and in and out of the bath and in all kinds of lifting for 15 years. Fifteen years. But then when I came here this was not acceptable to the service provider. I was told its service provider's policy on these slings had changed because another person with a disability had died as a result of using the sling. This website [http://www.hse.gov.uk/press/2011/coi-w-newportcc.htm] gives details.

Bruce: Yes, the technology in that sling was clearly insufficient.

Peter: Of course. And if it was shown to me that it was dangerous in the same kind of way then I'd have to have a new sling. But what I'm wanting to say is that I am very sensitive to being standardised—the sling is just an example. I guess it is also a matter of feeling in charge of my own life.

Bruce: So you're saying that's the issue here; that the changes to your life when you move out of independent living to a new facility with on-site supportive assistance need to be fully negotiated. And I guess you'll say that that also needs 'empathy' and a willingness to ignore stereotypes.

Peter: It's a matter of respect and being respected. With our concern for safety—I'm not denying the need for taking due care—we need to be careful we don't standardise people with disabilities.

Bruce: Or standardise managers as 'merely bureaucrats' who standardise people by rules?

Peter: I guess so. But I can't go home at night. People who live with the kinds of disability my body makes for me want to be looked at and respected on an individual basis.

Bruce: So you are taking the role here of advocate for disability not just criticising out of self-interest?

Peter: I hope so. For instance. As I have thought about my worries I remember that I felt really hurt that they wouldn't even let the sling I had used for 15 years be tried out so they could see how it worked. Now that was insensitive. After all, the day before moving in here I had been using the sling. And to refuse to see how it worked seemed to me to be saying that my life up until then somehow didn't count, at least not in terms of their management of my disability. Well that's wrong. They should not assume I am going to reinvent myself by coming to a new place.

Bruce: So this is Dr Peter Gibilisco, Disability Consultant, giving advice then?

Peter: Yes, and I'm not ashamed to take that role even if it is on a *pro bono* basis. I spent many years studying sociology and economics. I'm not completely unaware of management theory.

Bruce: That was an important part of your reflection on stereotyping wasn't it?

Peter: That is right. Think about it this way. It was not just the sling. As you've said, I'm usually a pretty optimistic fellow. You have to be if you are going to tackle life with this condition. You're up against what I call the medical model.

Bruce: You better explain that.

Peter: People with disabilities are first, presumed and believed to be medically inferior, which then becomes society's systematic norm—they are simply a cost—and that leads to cumulative disadvantage. It involved a complete rearrangement of the technology and equipment I have been using and which has helped keep me going for many years. Then, all of a sudden, the equipment that I was using did not meet the organisational safety standards for people with disability. As I suggested. It's as if something in the standardisation process wants me to forget just how much I coped before I came here and how. And to put it in pure materialistic terms: such a move to standardise disability has cost me a lot of money and created a bit of emotional turmoil.

Bruce: So, you are somewhat surprised by what you have encountered. I guess you have known all about it from your studies of sociology and economics. The kinds of hands-on 'lack-of-empathy' can get under your skin. So let's try to look at what needs to be considered for a person like your-self, who has to make the transition from relatively inde-pendent living—with outside support coming to your house—to supported living which needs to develop struc-tured 'empathy' to enhance a resident's genuine independ-ence when most day-to-day household affairs are taken care of.

Peter: I was first told about the house when I first applied for an increase in my Disability Service Register [DSR]. This house presented as a possible alternative to an increase in the DSR. This seemed a good option to me at the time since re-quirements for a DSR were strict and the facility promises comprehensive care and oversight.

Bruce: So you could also say that as your condition pro-gressed there were other constraints like pension and health benefits which were tightened and made the move somewhat more attractive?

Peter: Yes, I've been trained to see the flow-on effects of changes to regulations. People in my situation need others to remind them of these changes to the legal requirements.

Bruce: What do you mean by comprehensive care and oversight?

Peter: I'm referring to disability service provision. It has to do with the way a facility must present itself to the community it serves.

Bruce: Yes I recall reading your critique of the State Disability Plan. You've said that it is full of rhetoric that gives a good impression, but in actual day-to-day delivery there are hurdles. Are we dealing with something similar here?

Peter: Yes I think so. I have thought a lot about this. Don't get me wrong. The plan has an impact on independent living and also upon supported living. There are things that worry me. How do I make my voice heard without being misunderstood?

Bruce: It's not easy communicating and making your needs known when your muscles don't let you talk as clearly as you would like.

Peter: Exactly. I will have difficulties communicating with anyone let alone the management. How will they reckon with the fact that I am a PhD? I'm not a person with a cognitive disability and it would be unfair to stereotype me as one.

Bruce: So you feel in a bit of a bind, then? Your speech is now very slurred.

Peter: Sadly, yes. And when you want to stand up for yourself you don't want to give the impression that everything is wrong.

Bruce: Keep going. You've done a lot of thinking about this.

Peter: I'm pretty clear why I'm not happy. I feel as if I haven't been listened to.

Bruce: As you say your condition makes it hard for you to put into words why you are unhappy.

Peter: Exactly. That's why this interview format is helpful. I've had to think a lot about why I am worried and to check myself that I am not just over-reacting. But I'm not. I know I'm rather selfish at times. And yes, there's a management issue about dealing with people with my qualifications who want to speak up, let alone with my condition. And when you are running a place like where I am there has to be some kind of standards. But my problem is that I feel as if I am stereotyped.

Bruce: There's a wide range of people to be cared for. I guess there's not too many PhDs who are being cared for in these kinds of facilities. I guess there will also be those with cognitive and learning problems.

Peter: Exactly. And it's not that I'm wanting empathy only shown to me. I've got to show it too I guess. You've got to have standards and safety and things like that. But I've been used to living on my own for 21 years and using the sling for 15 of those years. And I had to manage my own life in different ways from what is now required. There were things I found worked for me when I was living in my own place, before I came here. And I know that my condition is progressive, so that the basic methods of lifting me and what I can and can't do will change.

Bruce: So this interview you've got me to have with you is to explain that you feel like you've been standardised. A bit like a MacBurger. We touched on that in sociology: McDonaldisation it was called. Standardisation in hamburgers. And you are saying it feels like that at times here.

Peter: Yes. Exactly. Management these days seems to have a similar standardised approach towards all types of disability. I can appreciate that a place needs standards but one of the standards must also be to listen or, in my case, take time to listen to what it is I am trying to say. Yes, it's difficult. And I wasn't the easiest person to communicate with before my speech was slurred. But if I said to the management that I felt as if I had been stereotyped in a negative way they might think I was just criticising because I was feeling sorry for myself.

Bruce: And are you?

Peter: What?

Bruce: Feeling sorry for yourself?

Peter: To some extent yes. I guess. But I want to point out that my disability is very different from that of others who live here. And I'm not just concerned about me. The sling issue has a flow-on effect to others, like support workers. So it is not just my personal needs here. I know that.

Bruce: One last thing. In one of your *OLO* pieces you discuss the mobility and your friendship with Rob of Frankston

Radio Cabs, your Maxi-Taxi driver. You are obviously concerned that those involved with caring for the disabled give due recognition to the need for people to move around. The concept of mobility needs to be opened up doesn't it?

Peter: When disability is viewed in terms of the medical model 'mobility' is understood in a very restrictive way. I'm wanting a shift towards a more feasible social model. How could I ever say that a person is no good, unless they are physically mobile? But if the medical model prevails that is what tends to happen at the expense of what I would call the perspective from a social model of mobility.

Bruce: Sociology has its own understanding of social mobility. And I guess the availability of computers, let alone wheelchairs, keeps you going, helps you to keep on pushing. I hope this interview also does that.

Peter: The coffee machine is over there; just help yourself to a cappuccino!

Where is the dignity in 'my future, my choice?'

Part 1

The disease was progressing severely, but nothing could equip me for the extreme loss of control of my life I was about to face in SSA. Sure, because of very slurred speech, I have difficulties communicating with management, but they should reckon with me as someone who is qualified (I do have a PhD and have studied sociology, economics and management). And if they are not taking my opinions into consideration, then they should know they are making me feel as if I am a person with a cognitive disability. I am very supportive and sympathetic of many clients in this house who have cognitive disabilities, but I am not one.

I am also supportive and sympathetic of the workers. They need to be encouraged to take the views of clients—in this case like myself—into account. One of the major reasons prompting me to decide to move to this new place had to do with my personal well-being. It was no longer safe for me to live on my own. This was basically due to the fact that DHS had held back my DSR, throughout my years of necessity for adequate support, that is, never have my cries for more support been totally accepted. But the last two years I had consistently and logically pleaded with DHS for an increase in my DSR. And during these two years, my disease had progressed severely, also, in part, as a result of the emotional turmoil created through insufficient care.

Basically, DHS would give me $69 000 to cover all of my care. At the time, I was wanting to increase my DSR by approximately $30 000, which would ensure further care on top of the customary care of morning and evening service, alleviating my vulnerability.

Although I have done a lot with my life, DHS still seemed to be opposed to my request for an increase in DSR even though, at least in terms of the rhetoric, 'mutual obligation' is the current political buzz word.

One of my major problems is the situation I now face in having to deal with casual staff. During the last two years when I lived on my own in Dandenong, I was in charge and managing the employment of caregivers in a direct way. One day, a few years ago, my main support worker was feeling under the weather. And on such short notice we needed to come up with an adequate replacement. I had heard good reports about this service provider, however, they provided me with a support worker whom I found to be very inadequate due to their inability to understand my speech. Recently, at Dunblane, casuals from the latter service provider have reappeared on my horizon.

One thing prompting the move to shared-support accommodation was my need for 24-hour care. I was being left on my own, and thus highly vulnerable, in between the regular times of care. One day, before I moved, I fell to the side of my wheelchair. The same thing happened on another occasion as I will explain below. But because of the restrictions on my support, I was left in an alarming position.

Recently, on a Friday night I received confirmation that my new DSR was approved. This proved to be a lifesaving matter in so many ways.

Just consider: one day, at around 8.00 pm the staff came to my room to deliver mail and they found me half out of my chair lying on the floor. I had fallen into that position an hour earlier. It left me in a position where it was impossible to reach the buzzer and here I was vomiting and yelling for one hour. I had just finished dinner.

In other words: I know very well what care I need. I am all too aware of the vulnerability of my situation. I just hope my new DSR level can now ensure a better level of safety.

Recently, at about 2.00 am in the morning, I was in a very uncomfortable sleeping position in bed, and I called by buzzer. No one turned up. I heard the next morning, that those on duty could not find my room key to come and assist me. Later that day, my father came to visit and straightaway he looked at me and asked if I was OK. He could see I was not. Then, of course, I ask him the same question. It was strange of him to turn up so suddenly. Then he told me that he received a call from staff the previous night, informing him of the situation, and mentioning that they will call him back if they are unable to access my room. But since he received no further calls, he got worried and came to visit me. This was very irresponsible, especially when they had already contacted him, a 75-year-old, at two in the morning! And, anyway, why had the casual staff not been properly informed about the location of the keys?

As I said, I know what I am talking about. Things have got to change. A new attitude is needed to face the reality of caring for those with disability. I hope this straight-from-the-shoulder piece can help those who should be thinking about these matters.

Part 2

In this article I take an autobiographical approach. It follows on from my account of previous dramas. I'm sorry to report incidents that have caused me immense pain, with physiological and psychological suffering that is unbearable and borders on torture.

Of course, it is easier for those providing services to standardise disability. The manager must remain in control, although standardising the way in which services are delivered causes serious difficulties for those who are cared for and also for carers. A person's real-life situation needs to be taken into account.

Having a disability does not necessarily mean that you are mentally impaired. Service providers of not-for-profit services seem to want to standardise disability to make it more amenable to organisational processes, which can then distrib ute work tasks according to an economically-oriented calculus.

Let me provide an example from my real-life experience that occurred on Tuesday evening, 19 March, 2013. This is an account of another incident when, once more, I fell out of my wheelchair.

It was just after dinner. I needed to empty my bladder, and as usual, my carers set me up in the appropriate way. But in so doing I slumped out of my chair, falling to its side. After waiting five minutes for the staff member to return, I decided to try to make myself a little more comfortable by moving a bit. But that movement had the opposite effect—my body involuntarily flung me forward and ... crack. My hip was broken.

The staff member arrived 30 seconds after this happened. I was in great pain and finally managed to convey to them that they should ring for an ambulance to take me to the hospital.

I repeatedly requested that I be taken to a private hospital as I had private medical insurance coverage. But due to my slurred speech and being in a lot of pain they had very little chance of understanding what I was trying to say.

They brought me to the Dandenong Hospital where I was X-rayed and my broken hip was discovered. They gave me pain relief and I felt more comfortable for an operation the next morning.

The operation was successful. But my major problem with what was administered concerns the drugs: I was put on an eight-hourly regime of two tablets of Valium and one of Endone. And I have a history of hallucinating with such a high dosage. My issue, at this point, is that I was not properly told the dosage of these medicines.

My hallucinations were very severe and were of incidents in which, as with terrorist attacks, I imagined my life was under threat. Please try to put yourself in such a situation before you laugh at me. It sounds ridiculous but it was extremely difficult for me to get over the emotional turmoil that was created by these terrifying hallucinations.

My real need is to exit this place where I have no control over my own life. The people making decisions for me are repeatedly making standardised decisions that leave out the most important factor—my true needs. This has been a recurrent aspect of the last few months that I've lived here, and the troubles I have had to confront.

It has become so difficult for me to express myself and to get my needs identified. Writing as I am doing now is my only way of communication for these issues. Due to my disability, I am not in a position to freely communicate even on paper. If the support worker is not used to my speech then they have to wait as I reply to their question with my typing speed that sometimes can't go faster than one word a minute. This is why I require a primary carer with 24-hour care. If incidents similar to those I have recounted occur, the carer would know my preferences and my medical history and would be aware of what I truly need. For example, they would direct me to a private hospital since they would know about my private medical insurance cover, and would also be able to oversee the medication given to me.

Part 3

To provide me with a move from shared-support accommodation to an individual support package—as I already have found accommodation that fits my requirements, and suits my needs—will allow me to be more independent and to fulfil my academic research in a more reasonable way. That is, with an individual support package, I will be able to have the constant and fulfilling methods of care that are needed.

I lived on my own for more than 21 years and then moved to shared-support accommodation as it seemed more appealing at the time. But in reality, it has created horrifying situations for me due to inadequate methods of care and standardised policies by the service providers. Now that I have accommodation in a more individually suited place, Department of Human Services does not want to give me a return to an individual support package. The inadequacies of my life are not helped by those at DHS who fail to see the big picture: that is, I would be helped out immensely from such a move, plus this would have a flow-on effect within the disability sector, by opening up another opportunity in SSA for, hopefully, a better-suited individual. In addition to this, another extreme problem arises, in that I cannot afford to live here when considering it as a social space with economic room to move. That is, the service provider charges me $535 per fortnight in rent and I get a pension of $875 per fortnight. This leaves me with a disposable income of $340 per fortnight, and with that money I need to buy my own soaps, shaving materials and medicines.

I have been able to find suitable alternative accommodation through the help of a close friend. However, I am unable to take up this opportunity because my current individual support package is insufficient for me for the 24-hour care that I need. The costs of the move can be offset to a certain degree, as I can significantly reduce these costs through direct employment. It will give me the chance to employ, administer, manage and pay the taxes of better-suited support workers. Direct employment also allows me to choose my own support workers, with no administration costs, who can become familiar with my care and flexible needs. There is also the opportunity that I shall bring to society as a person with a severe disability and a PhD who has social inclusiveness as a priority. All in all this cannot be achieved because of the inability of DHS to provide me with sufficient funding.

Also, direct employment would allow me to use my 20 years of post-secondary school training, especially my degree in accounting for administration and some systematic management issues. This is without mentioning my PhD in Sociology, which covered social-scientific subjects like Disability Studies, Political economics and Sociology. It is these social-scientific subjects that have allowed me to see the complexities of care and its management for people with severe disabilities. There is no doubt that my qualifications and knowledge of my disability supports are required to fulfil my life.

Therefore, I ask the question: who is best to administer and manage my supports, myself or a manager of a service provider who is far less academically qualified than myself, and has little awareness of my diverse needs while being restricted by the service providers' standardised policies and procedures concerning disability. It is my opinion that DHS, as well as the service provider, has underestimated the care required to look after me safely. For example, in the shared-support accommodation house, I am only receiving six hours of intensive support and for the rest of the time I have to ring the buzzer for somebody who is free. This is not what I require as I have on many occasions had a 30-minute wait for a staff member to come in. Such a wait caused me a lot of damage; similar experiences of negligence have dramatically added to my medical problems.

Works Consulted

Gibilisco, P (2004b) 'Is the Victorian government trying to avoid helping people in need?', On Line Opinion, February 16, 1-2, http://www.onlineopinion.com.au/view.asp?article=18 82.

Gibilisco, P. (2013), 'Where's the dignity in my future, my choice', *On Line Opinion,* 12 March 2013. Page 1–2, retrieved from http://www.onlineopinion.com.au/view.asp?article=14 782&page=2.

Gibilisco, P. (2013), 'Standardising disability', *On Line Opinion,* 05 April 2013. Page 1, retrieved from http://www.onlineopinion.com.au/view.asp?article=14 874.

Media Player (2008), Feedback comment to 'Itches and scratches—living with disability', *On Line Opinion,* 8 April 2008 4:56:42 PM, Page 1, retrieved from http://forum.onlineopinion.com.au/thread.asp?article= 7127&page=1.

CONCLUSION

This book consists of a discussion of dominant political ideas and their effect on social policy. Most political ideas today are dominated by what is commonly referred to as neoliberalism, and with what some left-leaning neoliberals call the third-way. But when we add social democracy to the list, we become aware of the appearance of a serious social dilemma. This book has been written because these policy developments are very important for how disability is understood and the outcomes of which have a decisive impact in employment, education and service provision.

By looking at the dominant political approaches, we are confronted by their key ideas, and their attitudes to themes such as the NDIS. This, then, may help us to think critically and more responsibly respond with pragmatic sensitivity to what is shaping the future of the disability sector.

In the first chapter, we looked at key themes that help us give greater attention to the need for a just society that is inclusive of people with disabilities. This is needed to improve the structure of our society in a basic way. That is, our progress as a society is defined by our progressive social thought. Due to an underlying neoliberal commitment the structure of our society is very often overlooked and proposals for change are put in the 'too hard basket'. This may be a hard thing to achieve due to a dominant neoliberal political structure. But trouble is, when we combine the medical model and the social model politically, we end up with a form of social dilemma for people with physical disabilities. The social model is a must in today's society. It allows people with physical disabilities to expect that their own future will be within society rather than outside it.

In the second chapter, I introduced neoliberalism. Basically this provides for the downfall of most progressive and pragmatic social policy. Neoliberals do not believe that social policy should be the responsibility of government, believing instead that the goods of social policy can be justly and equitably distributed through private hands, which effectively promotes the idea of a house built on sand.

The third-way is simply neoliberalism with a smiley face. That is, it is simply neoliberalism with a sprinkling of ideas co-opted from social democracy. But, its foundation is individualistic neoliberalism, nevertheless. Everything today, it seems, must have outcomes that provide for equilibrium. And also with the third-way there is a chance that social democratic outcomes can provide appropriate and just social outcomes. Social democracy is based on the idea of collective equal outcomes, whereas neoliberalism is based on the idea of individualism, which means every man for himself.

The next chapter highlighted how education has an impact on people with severe disabilities. I have mainly focused on my own situation where I have gained a great deal from education but, after achieving so much, I am left to ask: 'Where has it got me?' For sure, I am very talented, and able to write articles, but for whom and what purpose? Therefore, has education just provided me with a false expectation?

The next chapter looked at employment for people with disabilities. Among the general questions are those concerning stereotyping. The stereotypes are usually formed from what I have called the biomedical model, which has a very strong impact on the delivery of employment to people with disabilities. For example, there is this response to one of my *On Line Opinion* articles regarding employment in the disability sector: 'Having interviewed Peter for a temporary job, his disabilities made it difficult to employ him despite his insights and contacts.' This is the major reason for my disappointment in the not-for-profit disability and employment sectors. As you may know, there are great advances in the education sector concerning people with disabilities, but this has not been followed through in the employment sector.

The chapter on service provision looked again at personal struggles, with a system that has never acted in my favour. It looked critically at the Victorian State Disability Plan and then examined in an overall way how service provision becomes focused on standardisation and efficiency. Then, I looked at the mutually beneficial outcomes for people with severe physical disabilities, and raised again the importance of understanding employment and service provision in terms of synergy. Some ideas about how these important aspects of policy can be improved were included.

In Chapter 7, I adopted an interview format to get my message across. This outlines the struggles and barriers to shared-support accommodation, especially concerning people with physical disabilities but without any intellectual disabilities. This matter was raised gradually over a one-and-a-half-year period, giving rise to serious independence issues concerning control over my own life.

What are the general lessons from this journey? Among the many more specific analytical points and policy issues, there is one overriding principle: that the approach to disability should mainly be to empower people with disabilities. One sure method of doing so is to allow them to have control over their own lives.

I conclude with the words of Jenny Cooper (2006):

> We continue to stay in denial about who we are and still succeed as a nation. Disability is a part of what we are. Inclusion would acknowledge that. Destiny may one day lead us there. Or there's always revolution!

www.ingramcontent.com/pod-product-compliance
Lightning Source LLC
Chambersburg PA
CBHW031459270326
41930CB00006B/162